Gut Wisdom

UNDERSTANDING *and* IMPROVING *your* DIGESTIVE HEALTH

By

ALYCE M. SOROKIE

NEW PAGE BOOKS
A division of The Career Press, Inc.
Franklin Lakes, NJ

GUT WISDOM
EDITED BY JODI BRANDON
TYPESET BY EILEEN DOW MUNSON
Cover design by Cheryl Cohan Finbow
Printed in the U.S.A. by Book-mart Press

To order this title, please call toll-free 1-800-CAREER-1 (NJ and Canada: 201-848-0310) to order using VISA or MasterCard, or for further information on books from Career Press.

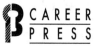

The Career Press, Inc., 3 Tice Road, PO Box 687,
Franklin Lakes, NJ 07417
www.careerpress.com
www.newpagebooks.com

Library of Congress Cataloging-in-Publication Data

Sorokie, Alyce M.
    Gut wisdom : understanding and improving your digestive health / by
Alyce M. Sorokie.
        p. cm.
    Includes bibliographical references and index.
    ISBN 1-56414-753-3 (pbk.)
    1. Gastrointestinal system—Diseases—Popular works. 2. Gastrointestinal
system—Diseases—Alternative treatment. 3. Indigestion—Popular works. 4.
Indigestion—Alternative treatment. 5. Medicine, Psychosomatic. I. Title.

RC817.S66 2004
616.3´3--dc22

2003064395

Disclaimer

This book is based on the research, experience, and opinions of the author. If symptoms persist, always check with the Wisdom of your Gut and with your doctor.

To Laura Ruby —————————

I have tremendous gratitude for your

help on this project.

You transformed my vision

into a reality.

A hug and a smooch to you, my friend.

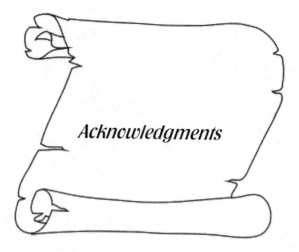

Acknowledgments

Very special thanks to Laura Ruby for generously editing and organizing my work. You cemented my pile of bricks. Thanks to Niambi Jaha Echols—my "book birthing coach." You were one of the angels nudging and pushing me to spread the word and get my message out. Thanks to Joan Epstein, Kari Schieble, Pam Gearhart, Dr. Gabrielle Frances, and Bob Condor for your discriminating eagle eyes, open hearts, and encouragement. Additional thanks to Miriam Smith, Angie Becerra, Ardath Berliant, Diane Valletta, and Kristin Amondsen for offering your computer-savvy and editing skills to this project. Also, warm acknowledgment to my dearest pal, Diane Cistaro, who phoned me daily during the process of writing this book. You were my very own cheerleader—even at times when I didn't want one. Thanks to Nora Harold and Carrol Chaiken for their spiritual counseling and assistance in helping me to transform my old beliefs about the difficulty of the pursuit of being published.

My gratitude to Career Press for seeing the wisdom and potential within my book and creating a great opportunity. Thanks to Mom for believing that I could do this as well as for embodying me with alternative health before it was called "alternative." Dad, though you have been watching me from the "other side" for the past 28 years, I have a "gut" feeling that you had a finger in this project. I cherish you for the challenges, the lessons, and bestowing this mission. Thanks to all of my clients who have also been my teachers. Together, we have explored gut-brain connections and have listened and answered your previously ignored gut distress. Finally, I acknowledge my inner gut wisdom, which continues to guide and direct me, even during times of resistance.

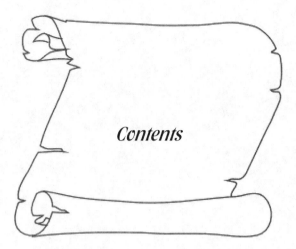

Contents

Preface		11
Introduction:	The Wisdom Within	15
Chapter 1:	The Gut Speaks	23
Chapter 2:	Grand Central Station: Know Your Friend	35
Chapter 3:	Death Begins in the Colon	49
Chapter 4:	Don't Kill the Messenger	59
Chapter 5:	Food: Friend or Foe?	65
Chapter 6:	The Gut Wisdom Diet: Building a Functional Relationship With Food	105
Chapter 7:	Gut Troublemakers	111
Chapter 8:	Gut Befrienders: Creating a Functional Relationship	123
Chapter 9:	Gut Wisdom Cleanse	151
Chapter 10:	What to Do	171
Conclusion:	Our Gut's Design	229
Appendix A:	Wisdom Quickies	231
Appendix B:	Standard Digestive Tract Tests	235
Appendix C:	Resources	239
Bibliography		243
Index		247
About the Author		255

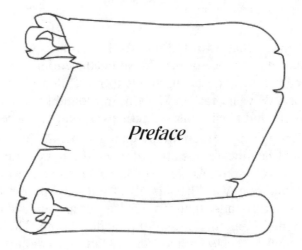

Preface

My life's mission was conceived at a very early age. I was raised by parents who were both mired in the dark ages and light years ahead of their time. In the 1950s, my father had one of the first health food stores in Chicago, well more than a decade before it was a "groovy" thing to do. I was raised on fruits, vegetables, and unadulterated whole grains while everyone around me dined on hamburgers, French fries, and colas. Junk foods were forbidden. Doctors, antibiotics, "sick" days—none of these were a part of my family's vocabulary. On the rare occasion when we did get sick, my parents used herbs and vitamins to strengthen our immune systems and heat packs and various water therapies—including the dreaded enema—to detox our systems and help our bodies do what they do best: *heal.*

Needless to say, I did not brag about my father's profession. Then, when I was 20 years old, the unthinkable happened: My 60-year-old father passed away from colon cancer, and I inherited the health food store. As customers came in and heard the news of his death, they were saddened and bewildered, and they wondered aloud how their "guru" could have died so young. Didn't eating yogurt and drinking distasteful green health drinks give you the license to live at least as long as the hundred-year-old Hunzas?

I was also saddened and bewildered and unable to answer their questions—or mine. How did this happen? How could my father be taken from this world so early, and by the very disease he seemed most prepared to fight? *What did my father do wrong?*

Michael Sorokie did not open a health food store because he was a free-spirited, tie-dye wearing, ultra-progressive hippie. Just the opposite: He was an uptight, hard-working, meat-and-potato-eating, right-winged truck mechanic. What attracted him to the business wasn't a change of heart as much as a change of health. An unconventional doctor had used herbs, supplements, and healing foods to miraculously cure my father's urethra cancer 30 years earlier. With his newfound knowledge, my father wanted to help and teach others. And he was quite a success.

Yet, although my father totally changed his attitude toward food, medicine, and healthcare, his attitude toward emotional expression was another story. Nowadays we get copious opportunities to work through anger, hurt, and grief with the support of self-help groups and therapists (even family and friends) that can help us accept, understand, and integrate the pain, disappointments, and tragedies of life. These things were not as prevalent in the 1950s and 60s. My father, as did many men of his time, kept his feelings tightly bottled up within him. The only feeling he seemed able to express was anger. And my father was *angry*. He was angry when he spoke, when he ate, when he worked. He was *marinated* in rage. My father, in his anger, would often grip his stomach area and shout, "This is making my gut sick!"

Despite his temper, my father's second bout with cancer, 30 years later, came on unexpectedly—who expects it? Seeing my father—this angry, seemingly invincible man, filled with a cantankerous spirit, yet strangely sensitive to the needs of his customers—doubled over with pain made *me* sick to my stomach. As the illness progressed, my father finally gave in and saw a conventional medical doctor for an official diagnosis. Initially, he needed a colostomy just to help relieve the discomfort of the growing malignancy. This was news we all wanted to deny, but my father's pain wouldn't let us.

Cancer, medical doctors, a colostomy, my dad—a nightmare. Within six months, he had passed on.

Soon after my father's death, I was consumed with questions: Didn't he eat well enough? Was it heredity (since then an aunt and cousin both suffered with, and beat, colon cancer)? Was it just his "time" to go? Or was all that pain and anger literally eating him up? Could emotional issues affect the digestive system? Could the mind actually alter the gut's basic processes? Could we learn something from our symptoms? Could changing our attitudes change our gut? Could the gut's health—or lack thereof—actually affect the choices we make?

As my desire to understand my father's death grew, so did my study of nutrition, massage therapy, various body/mind therapies, and my dear friend, colon therapy (a close cousin of my childhood enema). I began to integrate the scientific and the esoteric, the medical and the spiritual, knowing that within all these could lie the key to digestive health. I studied colon therapy and interned with a doctor whose specialty was helping very sick patients. There, I saw how dietary changes, vitamins, internal cleansings, colon therapy, lifestyle changes, and attitude shifts helped many a "Lazarus" rise. I saw severe arthritic conditions subside, neurological conditions reverse, debilitating digestive problems shift, and lists of chronic health problems disappear.

I closed the health store and began to work in alternative health centers, eventually opening my own clinic more than a decade ago, while continuing my studies in body/mind healing modalities. I was amazed over and over again by the healings I witnessed and was a part of. I saw unhealthy, congested, toxic digestive and eliminative systems get healthier and more robust. I also saw some clients go back to their old ways of eating and drinking, thus sabotaging their newfound health. I was curious about this.

I was also curious about some of the clients on whom I would perform abdominal massage and colonics. During their sessions, strong emotions surfaced. Memories of a mother's anger or the sadness around childhood sexual abuse, or sometimes just a pure sense of anxiety, would wash over my clients and then wash away, leaving them more calm, more peaceful. I began to notice that clients would often have a very bloated belly during or after traumatic times such as a death in the family, financial problems, divorce, and other struggles, as if they were "armoring" themselves against their pain. Sometimes, their guts' symptoms seemed to mirror what was going on for them emotionally. I also realized that, not only did I have to advise my clients about fiber and water intake, diet, and supplement changes, but I also had to acknowledge some very real emotional issues that lay behind much of my clients' physical distress.

My father's journey was a gift to me, because it instilled the desire to explore and understand the dynamics of the body and mind in digestive and eliminative health and illness. The use of healthy diet and herbs, vitamins, enemas, and so forth helped me to trust natural remedies. His death, however, led me to journey within, to investigate my own unexplored emotional business, to move beyond the physical to the metaphysical (our thoughts, emotions, and spirit). With my upbringing and formal education in nutrition, I understood the importance and impact of a healthy diet. If you eat enough fiber and drink enough water, the gut can generally be a wonderful companion. And if genetics predispose a person to a rumbling, cranky gut, dietary and lifestyle changes can often help. But what I've come to learn is that, if you're eating the right foods, exercising, and getting enough rest, and your gut is still "speaking" with symptoms, then one must look to beyond the body. The foods we eat, our emotions, our thoughts, our words, our genetics, our deepest beliefs all intertwine and affect our gut's health—or lack of it.

A Little Deal With God

From my father, I learned that eating the healthiest foods is often not enough. *You also need healthy attitudes and healthy emotional processing.* This curiosity soon led me to a certification in the Hendricks Body/Mind Centering Process. I've also studied Hakomi, Focusing, the ancient art of Mayan abdominal massage, Reiki, and many other body/mind modalities—each of which emphasized the need to *honor* the body and *listen* to its wisdom. I continue my education in nutrition at Clayton Naturopathic College, an institution whose philosophy about nutrition and the body is as open as my own. At first, I thought I was simply augmenting my work at my health center, but I soon realized that I was learning methods that just might help prevent what happened to my father from happening to others. Maybe I was also trying to make a little deal with God: If I helped as many people as possible, could I turn my father's tragedy into a legacy? Could I help others understand that healthy emotional processing is as vital to overall health as diet and exercise?

I began offering Gut Wisdom workshops around the Chicago area and the Midwest. I invented an herb-filled, comforting pillow I fondly call the Belly Buddy that can be warmed and used to soothe an aching gut, a creation that has received enthusiastic write-ups in periodicals from *Spa* to *Today's Chicago Woman* to the *New York Daily News*. I've also shared my wisdom through dozens of newspaper interviews and television appearances to get the word out about the Gut Wisdom within each of us.

During the last 15 years I have questioned myself: What the heck are you doing, girl? You spend your days providing nutritional counseling and colonics and your weekends facilitating Gut Wisdom workshops that focus on bellyaches!?! You talk about bodily functions that most parents caution their children *never* to mention in polite company. Aren't you a bit of a kook? Sometimes I answer back, "Yep, this is pretty taboo stuff!" But most of the time I feel gratitude for the opportunity to witness people freeing themselves from years of discomfort and pain with the magic of diet, colonics, massages, intestinal cleansings, and simple *awareness.*

Awareness of what? Gut Wisdom, of course!

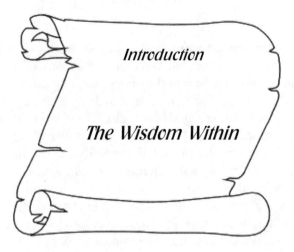

Introduction

The Wisdom Within

Judy was introduced to a "fabulous" new guy by some of her friends. Everyone thought he was perfect for her. And when Judy met him, she agreed that he did *seem* perfect: good-looking, smart, romantic, always saying the right things, and so on. But each time they met, Judy got a tight, painful knot in her gut, accompanied by nausea. When she shared this with her friends, they'd say, "It's all in your head" or "You must be scared of a good man." So she kept seeing the man and endured the wracking nausea—until she found out this "perfect" guy was married (a minor detail he'd failed to share with her). What did her gut know that her head didn't?

For more than 15 years, George has been plagued by nearly crippling gut discomfort. George has been unable to go out without fear that he might lose control of his bowels. He kept close to home and made sure he knew where the restrooms were in the stores where he shopped. His visits with friends were brief and fraught with anxiety and embarrassment. Feeling despair and pain, he didn't dare give up the few things that gave him comfort: wine, dairy foods, and chocolate. In a Gut Wisdom workshop, George had a profound realization: His debilitating gut distress began soon after his wife left him for another man. He felt "so out of control"— feelings his digestive and eliminative systems seemed to mirror with their "runaway" symptoms. He made the choice to let go of the betrayal and move on with his life. Soon after his important realization, George's symptoms became less severe, and George was less resistant to dietary and lifestyle changes that soothed his gut and, eventually, his heart. Was his gut expressing something he could not?

John came to me years ago complaining of chronic constipation. As a matter of fact, he would often use the phrase, "I'm stuck." He felt stuck in his life and in his job. He yearned to be something different, something "free," like a "ski bum." The truth was that John was making a six-figure income and enjoyed the money. He was also a perfectionist, always telling himself that he must do things "correctly," always chastising himself for his mistakes. And the more he punished himself, and the harder he drove himself, the more "stuck" he got—mentally and physically. It was only when John finally accepted the fact that he really didn't *want* to leave his job that he was willing to make a few attitude adjustments. Along with some changes in his diet, he learned how to deep breathe when he got stressed. He began to take walks when he was tempted to berate himself. John began to take extended ski trips so that he could be a ski bum—if only for a little while. As John gradually relaxed, so did his constipation. Was John's gut trying to tell him something?

Judy, George, and John are just three of the millions of Americans who suffer digestive and eliminative complaints such as indigestion, constipation, diarrhea, heartburn, and irritable bowel syndrome. Perhaps you are one of them. Every day at my healthcare center, Partners in Wellness, I see smart, successful, and talented people whose lives are being ravaged by digestive and eliminative illnesses. I've listened to their stories of suffering and pain, and, luckily, I've had the privilege of being a part of their stories of success and healing.

Are you one of millions of Americans who constantly ignore his or her own "gut instincts," such as the rock in your stomach that told you that your date was no good for you or the cramps that came with every visit from your brother? Later, when you experienced heartburn after that fast food you ate, you realized your gut was telling it like it is and that, yes, oh yes, yes: You *should* have listened.

The wisdom of your gut "knows" what you need. It is an inner knowing, a nonrational, nonintellectual, nonlinear way of knowing. It's your intuition, your inner antennae, and your truth-teller. It's the wisdom of the body that attempts to guide and direct you, to make you aware of the things you do to sabotage yourself and your gut's health.

It is time to become aware of, honor, and respect your gut's "voice" of guidance. Other cultures have long recognized the importance of the gut (belly). Cultures such as Indian, Chinese, Japanese, and African have held the belly as a point of access to spiritual power. In fact, some of these cultures have created methods—dance, t'ai chi, yoga—to help people learn how to honor and engage the gut as a source of wisdom and strength. Even in the West, our language refers again and again to the "power" and "wisdom" of the gut. For example, a "gutsy" person is a brave person. A flash of intuitive insight is called a "gut reaction" or "gut feeling." To "gut it out" is to be motivated and persistent.

The concept of body/mind unity is rooted in antiquity. The ancient Chinese Taoist sages viewed the body and mind as one interrelated whole. They believed that we not only digest and assimilate foods in our gut, but we also digest our *emotions* in our gut. If we repress, deny, or ignore these emotions, gut function is affected. Modern science is catching up with ancient wisdom. Even the most hard-nosed scientific researchers have been forced to acknowledge the body/mind connection when it comes to our health. It's a vicious cycle: Psychological stress plays a large role in creating or adding to the development of common gut ailments. This, in turn, adds to our stress, leading to more physical symptoms and compromising our immune system. When stress is not dealt with, when accompanying feelings are ignored or discounted, or when we hold ourselves back from experiencing life, the body revolts. Stress, long-held regrets, anger, and frustration can be major causes of irritable bowel syndrome, constipation, diarrhea, nausea, bloat, and more. Today's emerging interest in psychoneuroim-munology (the scientific study of the relationship between the brain and the body's immune system) is bringing ancient wisdom the scientific support it deserves.

Compelling new research has also shown that in each person's gut is a sophisticated network of nerve cells more extensive than that of the spinal cord—more than 100 million in the small intestine alone—called the enteric nervous system, or gut-brain (or second brain or abdominal brain; I will kindly call it the gut-brain). This primitive nervous system consists of networks of neurons, many of the same neurotransmitters found in the cerebral brain, and cells that nourish neurons, which are involved in immune responses. The vagus nerve connects the gut-brain and the cerebral brain, enabling both to send signals to each other and react to these signals. Researchers theorize that the cerebral brain can either slow down the gut-brain or over-stimulate it. Yet, though the enteric nervous system (gut-brain) is influenced by messages from our cerebral brains, it can direct and coordinate all our digestive, absorptive, and eliminative activities *without* input. The gut-brain can "sense" data, "process" information, and "act" independently from the brain proper. A new field known as neuro-gastro-enterology has emerged, joining together neuroscientists who study the brain and spinal cord with gastroenterologists who treat heartburn, chronic stomach pain, and diarrhea. Pioneers in this new field, such as Michael Gershon, M.D., have postulated that, because the enteric nervous system was designed to function independently, the gut-brain may be subject to its own "mental" illnesses, much as our topmost brain is.

Other researchers have emphasized that the nerve cells of the gut produce neuropeptides, powerful chemicals that communicate information from cell to cell. These affect our moods and all of our biological systems, including our immune system. Neuropeptides are a direct line of communication between our emotions and our bodies. (As much as 95 percent of the body's serotonin—believed to have a profound role in the creation of happiness—is made in the gut!) The gut is also a rich source of benzodiazepines, chemicals in the same family of psychoactive drugs as Xanax and Valium.

Because of all this cutting-edge research, some scientists now believe that the complex structure of the gut enables it to feel, learn, and remember and that the gut-brain can have as much to do with the "human condition"—happiness, sadness, hope, and despair—as the brain proper. Unlike thoughts in our heads, however, the gut's "thoughts" and "feelings" are often experienced as nausea, knots, butterflies, pulls, tension, bloat, constipation, diarrhea, or more severe symptoms. Unfortunately, we have been trained to discount these gut feelings. We often do everything we can to rid ourselves of these unpleasant sensations and symptoms without ever asking ourselves what they might mean.

Taboo No More: Have We Ignored Our Gut Wisdom for Too Long?

Putting the bowels (gut) in the closet and making believe they don't exist have lead many down the path of improper living, treating the bowel indiscriminately, and reaping the sad harvest in later years.

—Dr. B. Jensen,
Tissue Cleansing Through Bowel Management

In Chicago, I have a TV show on cable entitled *Gut Wisdom*. On a recent trip to the post office, the worker behind the counter said, "I saw you on TV the other night, and you were talking about...about...you know, about stuff down there...your gut and sorts...." I was reminded of and amused by our society's discomfort with guts and bodily functions. Amusing as it may be, however, this taboo against toilet talk has created some staggering statistics.

More than 70 million individuals have reported that they suffer from gastrointestinal problems, according to the U.S. Department of Health and Human Services. This epidemic of digestive and eliminative problems will not go away if we give in to our squeamishness and continue to ignore this vital subject. The colon—and the rest of the digestive and eliminative system—is one of the most neglected and forgotten parts of the body. *The key to gut health is listening to the gut and taking appropriate action.*

Consider this. In the United States:

In the 1950s, diverticulosis (a herniation of the large intestine's muscular lining) affected only 10 percent of adults aged 45 and older. In 1987, almost *50 percent* of the population was diagnosed with this disease. According to the Merck Manual, the most recent reports predict that *everyone* will be diagnosed with diverticulosis at some point after the age of 40.

▸ More than eight million people have complained of constipation, with many more attempting self-medication. More than 500 million dollars a year is spent on laxatives.

▸ Irritable bowel syndrome is the #1 digestive problem, rivaling the common cold in terms of medical costs and lost work hours.

▸ Every year, 100,000 colostomies are performed. This is a surgical procedure that requires the removal of a portion of the colon. Afterwards, one must eliminate wastes through an opening in the abdomen into a pouch outside the body. Sometimes colostomies are used temporarily to allow the gut to heal after intestinal surgery. In other cases, a colostomy is permanent.

▸ More than 70 million Americans suffer from digestive disorders. Of those Americans, 17.7 million have been diagnosed with ulcers.

▸ Hemorrhoid medication Preparation H is the fourth-largest-selling over-the-counter medication.

▸ Colorectal cancer will kill approximately 60,000 Americans this year, with another 125,000 new cases diagnosed. It is the second leading cause of death from cancer in the United States.

Can it be that ignoring your gut wisdom can lead to illness? I believe the answer is yes.

Pain can be a wonderful thing. Without pain, we could step on rusty nails or cut our hands and never realize anything is wrong until we see our feet or fingers turn red and mottled with life-threatening infection.

When a gut discomfort or illness strikes, apparently out of the blue, it can be a jolt. And if it is severe enough, it can stop us from carrying on as usual. This is possibly what the discomfort is meant to do. Inconvenient and distressing symptoms do, in fact, have a purpose. Symptoms are your gut's way of getting your attention. Your symptoms (pain, knots, butterflies, bloating, gas, constipation, nausea, and so forth) are the voice of the gut offering its guidance.

Our Responsibility

We can't choose our genetic make-up nor control the mysteries of the unknown. However, we can choose to become more aware of our thoughts and to honor our emotions and our attitudes. By addressing the stress in our physical, mental, emotional, and spiritual bodies—with lifestyle changes, foods, exercise regimens, thought and attitude adjustments, and other protocols that are addressed in this book—we can enrich our lives and the health of our guts. Remember the old saying: A fool is a person who does the same things over and over again, expecting a different result.

So, I am going to talk about things that might seem strange, gross, or "touchy-feely." I'm going to talk about what goes in our mouths and what comes out in the toilet (gasp!). I'm going to ask you to STOP and listen to the voice of your gut so you can learn how to benefit from its wisdom. And I will invite you to *befriend your gut* and reclaim yourself and your health.

I can't promise you *perfect* health, but if you follow the guidance in this book, you can:

> Discover how your emotions, your thoughts, and your attitudes affect your gut's health, and vice versa.

> Understand how your body's vital digestive and eliminative processes work.

> Learn ways to eat that will lessen gut pain and discomfort.

> Discover easy-to-use natural methods to prevent and soothe digestive and elimination ailments.

> Lose weight.

> ▷ Improve your overall health.

> ▷ Gain energy.

> ▷ Learn to listen to your gut's messages.

> ▷ Learn how building a relationship with your gut can put you back on the road to health.

I designed *Gut Wisdom* so that it can be used as a reference or as a journey. If you're looking to find remedies and protocols you can use immediately to treat a specific ailment, just turn to Chapter 10, where you'll find treatments for common gut issues such as constipation, irritable bowl syndrome, ulcers, and more. Or, if you'd just like to learn to eat better to prevent gut symptoms, turn to the Gut Wisdom Diet in Chapter 6. If you're more interested in taking things slowly, in learning how the gut affects the entire body and how the body affects the gut, you can read this book from beginning to end. There's no right or wrong way, as long as you get started.

So, are you sick and tired of being sick and tired? Then put your ear to your gut and listen for a while. It has something very important to tell you.

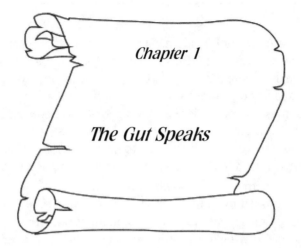

Chapter 1

The Gut Speaks

I get no respect.

—Rodney Dangerfield

Greetings. I am your gut. The funny thing about me is that you don't give me a thought unless you're having a problem of some sort. Say, you're bloated and you can't zip up your favorite jeans. Or you feel nauseous after you eat ice cream, or pizza, or broccoli, or practically anything else. Or you are sitting...and sitting...and sitting on the toilet and nothing is happening the way it's supposed to, or, on the flip side, you can't stop what's happening.

I, the gut, have become the root of lots of misery and discomfort for you. If only you could understand me and my language, you would know that I am your closest, most intuitive, wisest, and pretty much all-knowing friend.

I know how you have been living your life and what you need, desire, and feel. I know if you've been eating more potato chips than carrots and drinking more coffee than water. I know what stresses you out and what relaxes and soothes you. I know which people you should get close to and which people from whom you should run away (fast!). The problem is that you don't listen to me.

Somewhere along the way you got disconnected from the vital, sacred, wise part of you: *me*—your gut, your belly, your inner source of wisdom. Maybe your mother, father, or teacher told you too many times how you "should" or "shouldn't" feel. Maybe someone said that big girls and boys don't cry, don't scream, don't mourn. Maybe you learned a long time ago that our fast-paced society rewards people who talk about what they think, not about what they feel. Maybe you're too busy trying to squeeze 12 hours into eight to pay attention to me and give me what I need instead of stuffing me with fast food and alcohol.

But that's exactly why I've been calling to you. When I feel abandoned by you, I can become a pain. Literally. I might show up as bloat, gas, backaches, constipation, irritable bowel syndrome, diarrhea, hemorrhoids, anxiety, or depression. And if you still don't acknowledge me, I can speak loudly with diverticulitis, ulcerations, even cancer. Every thought and emotion has an affect on me. I get upset when you worry or get angry. I remember old hurts and painful physical and emotional experiences. I take in information even when your intellect doesn't notice.

You unconsciously shut me off when you take a shallow breath, eat poorly, or pop a pill in order *not* to feel certain emotions or physical discomforts. I nourish every inch of you. I try to guide you with all kinds of sensations. You try to flatten me with sit-ups, girdles, and tight belts. You say mean things: "This bloat is terrible, this bellyache is awful. Make it go away!"

Listen, I'm not bad. I'm just trying to get your attention. These painful signals I'm sending are good and life-promoting. I am working hard to regulate your well-being. The pain and discomfort are warnings, giving you a wake-up call so that you will *stop* and inquire, "What is really going on?" I want to be heard! I may need a change in diet. I may be telling you to stop and smell the roses...or the daisies...or the wheat grass. I may be telling you that it's time for you to start expressing those feelings that are eating *both* of us up. My voice may also be inviting you to address and heal those terrible hurts you have suffered, which you struggle to repress, which still run your life.

Some changes are simple ones; others may require much more courage, prayer, time, and love.

I am your friend, longing to reconnect with you.

—Your Gut

Have you ever noticed that you do not consciously control your digestion? Do you remember having butterflies in your stomach when you fell in love and intestinal cramps when you fell out of it? Ever follow a "gut feeling" about a situation and you were right on the mark? All these are functions of your gut-brain or enteric nervous system.

Yes, you have two brains! One is located in your skull and the other in your gut in the lining of your gastrointestinal system. Both brains originated during fetal development from tissues called the neural crest. One section turned into your central nervous system (brain and spinal cord), and the other developed into your enteric nervous system or second brain in your gut. These two brains are connected by a few thousand nerve fibers called the vagus nerve, with most of the nerve fibers coming *up from the gut* to the brain, so they can relay messages back and forth to each other.

Dr. Michael Gershon, researcher and author of *The Second Brain*, states, "nearly every substance that helps run the brain has turned up in the gut." The gut-brain has its very own supply of neurons, neurotransmitters, and neuropeptides, just as your cerebral brain does, which means that it can send and receive messages in the same way. The intriguing thing about the gut-brain is that it can operate on its own—like a free spirit, if you will—without any input from your other brain; it coordinates the process of digesting and eliminating food and absorbing nutrients without conscious thought. However, our two brains often act codependently. When one brain gets upset, so does the other. When your cerebral brain experiences stress, such as getting fired from your job or having an argument with your significant other, your gut may respond with cramping, nausea, or a bout of diarrhea.

Your gut-brain can also upset your other brain. Gut discomforts in the form of constipation, cramping, and irritable bowel syndrome can affect your cerebral brain by sending up messages of pain, altering your moods and your behavior.

Lines of Communication

There are several lines of communication that allow conversation between the cerebral brain and gut: the central nervous system, the autonomic nervous system, the enteric system, hormones called neuropeptides, and the energy systems.

Central Nervous System

The central nervous system—which consists of the brain and spinal cord—coordinates voluntary movement, translating your thoughts into electrical impulses that fire in your muscles. The central nervous system directs the muscles that help you pick up a fork, go for a walk, talk to someone, or perform any deliberate action. Your central nervous system also responds to your gut via impulses fired along the vagus nerve that connect cerebral brain to the gut-brain.

Autonomic Nervous System

The autonomic nervous system has two different types of nerves that perform different actions in the body: one that revs us up and the other that slows us down. In response to real or *perceived* danger and/or stress, the activating part of the autonomic nervous system, the *sympathetic nervous system*, revs us up by pumping out stress hormones such as adrenaline and cortisol. This increases our heart rate and blood pressure, muscle tension, hormone levels, metabolism, and brain activity. Breathing becomes shallow and rapid. Blood is shunted from the digestive tract, which slows digestion and elimination (which can result in indigestion, constipation, diarrhea, and irritable bowel flare-ups) and increases flow to the limbs to prepare us for "fight or flight." This is part of the reason why we experience that "sinking feeling" in our guts when we are afraid.

This "fight or flight" response to stress isn't necessarily bad; it enables us to respond to real danger and threats, such as running from a mugger. Unfortunately, we don't just experience racing hearts and a meltdown in our digestive and elimination system in response to real danger; we can experience it in response to *anything*. Anxious, fearful thoughts about unpaid bills, screaming children, car troubles, problems at work, and so forth can all trigger this "fight or flight" response. Our guts do not distinguish between real physical danger and perceived threats and stress.

However, we're not revved up all the time. In times of rest, the calming and restorative part of the autonomic nervous system, the *parasympathetic nervous system*, is working. This keeps our heart rate and blood pressure stable, keeps our breath slow and deep, and diverts blood back to the internal and digestive organs, allowing our body and gut to rest and heal.

Enteric Nervous System

The enteric nervous system can and does function autonomously, however normal digestive function requires communication links between this intrinsic system and the central nervous system (CNS). These links take the form of parasympathetic and sympathetic fibers that connect either the central and enteric nervous systems or connect the CNS directly with the digestive tract. Through these cross-connections, the gut can provide sensory information to the CNS, and the CNS can affect gastrointestinal function. Connection to the central nervous system also means that signals from outside of the digestive system can be relayed to the digestive system (that is, for example, the sight of appealing food stimulates secretions in the stomach).

Neuropeptide Chemical Messenger System

Neuropeptides are tiny protein molecules that are manufactured and secreted by our top brain, as well as our gut's brain, organs, and immune system.

Neuropeptide chemical messengers are a two-way communication system. They carry our emotions, attitudes, perceptions, and intellectual thoughts from the brain to the body and from the body to the brain.

Experiences of love or joy and fear or depression cause the cells in the limbic system (your brain's emotional processing center) to release neuropeptides to enter the bloodstream. Within a blink of an eye, these chemicals attach themselves to cells' receptor sites throughout the body—altering your body's physiology, so that each cell in your body responds to that emotion. Each emotion is transformed into a physical response, resulting in cellular changes throughout the entire body. Positive thoughts and feelings induce healthful physiological shifts, whereas negative ones have a detrimental effect. When feeling love, you experience feeling light, your heart feels open, and there is an obvious and very real sparkle in your eyes. How about the experience of anger? Your muscles are tight, your face may be flushed, and your stomach may ache.

Not only does the brain communicate through the neuropeptide system directly with the body, but, because the body manufactures these same chemicals, it is able to converse back to the brain.

Again, neuropeptides are not just present and manufactured in the brain, but also in our organs, immune system, and *throughout the gut*. What this means is that our entire body can, and often does, feel and express emotion. In fact, the entire digestive and elimination tract is filled with neuropeptide messenger chemicals, from the esophagus through the end of the gastro-intestinal system (rectum). Dr. Candace Pert, neuroscientist and author of *Molecules of Emotion*, implies that the gut has many neuropeptide messengers that make it a likely spot for us to "feel" a lot of strong feelings (that is, our "gut feelings").

Most importantly, messenger chemicals not only facilitate the two-way communication system between the brain and the gut, but also with the immune system. Actually, 70 to 80 percent of the body's immune cells reside in the gut. Research has shown that our emotional responses influence our immune function:

> "Grief, distress, fear, worry and anger are emotions which have horrible effects on the body's function. Researchers have discovered that these emotions cause the release of chemicals—neuropeptides. These potent compounds have a profound immune-suppressive action. Scientists have traced a pathway from the brain to the immune cells [and from the immune system to the brain] proving that negative emotions can stop the immune cells dead in their tracks.... Once this happens, harmful microbes or cancer cells can invade any tissue in the body."

> —Dr. Cass Igram,
> *Eat Right or Die Young*

Every feeling and thought we have creates a biochemical response within our body. By changing our mental state, what we eat, whether we exercise, and if we give and receive sufficient hugs, we have the power to influence the production of these chemical messengers with us.

Molecules, Schmolecules—What the Heck Does All This Mean?

▸ Our body and brain cannot be separated, as one always affects the other.

▸ Neuropeptides carry our hopes and dreams as well as our fears and concerns to every corner of our being.

▸ Our emotions, attitudes, and thoughts are all mirrored in the physiology of our body.

▸ Every thought and feeling create a biochemical response within our body. Some are health-promoting; other are detrimental.

▸ Production of neuropeptides can be influenced by our mental state and lifestyle choices.

▸ Your gut is in communication with you.

Energy System

Modern science has only begun to acknowledge the brain's influence on the body, and it has yet to embrace the idea that the body may have some influence on the brain. Yet Asian philosophers and medical practitioners have recognized the interconnectedness of the mind and body for thousands of years. The Asian belief system dictates that the gut does not simply digest and assimilate food, but also acts as the "seat" of our emotions. This ancient paradigm believes that each emotion is literally an expression of energy, and it has understood the undeniable affect our thoughts and emotions have on our health in general and on our gut health, specifically. Fortunately for us, Western medical thought is rediscovering this ancient wisdom. A case in point is the information we are presently learning about neuropeptides: The cells that create and carry emotion exist in our immune system.

Chi, qi, life force, soul, hara, prana—these are just some of the names given to energy, the life force that is central to our health and well-being. Through thousands of years of observation, study, and application, the discovery in China of 360-plus points throughout the body took place. These high-energy areas are found along pathways called meridians and are located within the muscles corresponding to particular physical and psychological functions and responses within the body. For example, anger affects the liver; holding on to toxic thoughts and attitudes affects the function of the large intestine; over-analyzing and obsessions will disrupt sleep patterns and cause a spleen imbalance. Research has shown that these points are "electrically charged" differently than that of the surrounding areas in the body. Additionally, endorphins ("feel good" chemicals) are released by the brain and body when these high-energy points are stimulated through the art of acupuncture or acupressure. This "flow of energy" is also affected by the foods we eat, exercise, and our ability to process emotions.

As does the circulatory system that delivers blood throughout your body, the meridian channels ensure that chi flows through the limbs and organs. Doctors of Chinese medicine believe that repressed emotions can block these channels and prevent the flow of vital energy required to keep the body in homeostasis balance. If our emotional disturbances can't find an outlet through healthy expressions and releases, they can collect in the gut. Consequently, these accumulated "imbalances" will contribute to a myriad of ailments, from lumps and tumors to constipation, gut irritations, headaches, and even heart disorders and kidney imbalances such as diabetes.

In my practice as a colon therapist and in my Gut Wisdom workshops, I've observed my clients as I taught them how to massage, breathe, and bring awareness to their guts using various techniques. They were often surprised at how feelings of sadness, grief, and anger emerged. These feelings were usually underneath symptoms of nausea, cramps, constipation, and diarrhea!

As it turns out, we don't just hold or repress those unpleasant negative feelings but also the positive feelings such as joy or love! Has anyone unexpectedly given you a public display of affection—and it felt so warm and validating? But maybe it was too embarrassing, and you just couldn't take it in. Processing pent-up feelings such as these are equally as important as the negative feelings. Deep-breathing awareness, massage, and other deeper body-mind techniques and therapies may facilitate a healthy release.

Gut Exploration Exercise

Spend a moment gently massaging your own belly, breathing deeply as you massage. Notice if there are any tense or tender areas that may be your own personal holding areas. You may be surprised at how the simple act of touch can cause the release of tension and emotion.

So, we can see that a bellyache may be your gut's way of trying to bring its processes to your conscious attention; it's trying to tell you something.

Can you imagine ignoring, discounting, or dismissing every thought you had? Yet many of us regularly ignore the "thoughts" of our bellies: the rumbles, butterflies, knots, cramps, or even disease. Our guts act in much the same way our cerebral brains do, processing information and inciting chemical riots that can cause us to dance with happiness or double over in pain. Considering the power and influence of the gut-brain, how can you afford to ignore it?

The Disconnection

Ironically, we are all too often educated out *of, rather than* into *awareness of the body.*

—Jean Houston

How did we get so far away from ourselves, from our own bodies, our guts, our gut wisdom? How is it that we now participate in the creation of symptoms, discomfort, and disease?

▸ **Puritanical Prudes**. In our society, there are certain spoken and unspoken "rules" governing our conversations and behavior. We are often taught not to talk about what happens in the bathroom at all; or if we do, it's only with a smirk and a snicker. Our lack of openness and knowledge about the workings of the gut sets us up for gut ailments.

▸ **Media**. Magazines, television, and advertisements constantly tell us that we don't have to pay attention to our gut's discomforts. We can pop a pill and move on. They convince us that our symptoms (our guts' voices) are simply inconveniences rather than important messages we need to listen to.

▸ **Gut Intruders**. Sexual abuse, rape, physical violence, and verbal and emotional abuse can cause one to shut down, numb out, repress, and ignore the gut's messages just to survive the sense of personal violation.

▸ **Other Disconnecting Traumas**. A difficult pregnancy, surgery, abortion, menstrual cramps, and other painful events often make us want to ignore sensations in our gut.

▸ **Intellectual Snobs**. As a society, we intellectualize and rationalize rather than follow our gut and listen to and trust our "gut feelings."

▸ **Lifestyle**. Our lives move so quickly and our schedules are so packed that there is little time for or interest in slowing down to listen to our inner voices of wisdom.

Building a Relationship

Yoo-hoo...your gut is speaking! Your gut is calling to be acknowledged, understood, and listened to. It's not creating bellyaches, pains, and discomforts just because it's bored and has nothing else to do. It's bloated because it wants to be *noticed*. It's cramping because it wants to be *heard*. Those irritating sensations, those horrible knots, the fiery gut, that creeping nausea—these are the tactics the gut uses to voice its wisdom in order for you to listen.

Cooperation between brain and gut is essential to maintain digestive and eliminative health. Chemical responses in your gut—due to the foods you eat and the lifestyle you live—are linked to your behavior and moods. Likewise, the emotions, thoughts, and attitudes you have are directly linked to chemical responses in your gut. Our thoughts and feelings may not be things we can see, but every thought or feeling creates a biochemical change right down to our cells, altering us physically.

Building any *functional relationship* is a process that involves listening, honoring the "voices" that are present, understanding the needs and wants, and embracing the discomforts as the messages they are. When you listen, honor, understand, and embrace, you create a relationship of ease, peace, and nourishment.

In a *dysfunctional relationship*, what often occurs are denial, avoidance, and repression. Instead of ease and peace, there is struggle. This struggle is accompanied by negative thoughts and attitudes, resistance, anxiety, anger, and frustration, which eventually will result in discomfort.

Karen, a 28-year-old woman, came to me after suffering with irritable bowel syndrome for four long years. Though she exercised every day and ate healthy foods, her constipation, diarrhea, and abdominal spasms could put her out of commission for days. I had a "gut feeling" that her condition might be related to an emotional experience, so I invited her to a Gut Wisdom workshop. At the workshop, she began to befriend her gut with deep-breathing exercises, massage, healing warmth, and just asking the gut what it needs or wants. Through these exercises and others, she made a realization and a connection that she had never made before. A little more than four years earlier, her fiancé died of a drug overdose. Her family, who didn't believe he was good enough for her, didn't support her in her grief and instead said things such as "This is for the best" and "Just move on." So Karen stuffed and denied her pain and tried to soldier through it, repressing her grief. A month later, her gut rebelled with irritable bowel syndrome. Armed with this new awareness, Karen sought the help of a grief counselor so that she could safely process the painful feelings that had been buried in her heart and sickening her gut. After three months of emotional processing and thorough counseling, her irritable bowel syndrome symptoms subsided.

Taking That First Breath

I began with "The Gut Speaks" purposefully. My intention is to invite you to develop a functional relationship with your gut—that abandoned part of you that is calling for your attention. You can keep running, but you can't hide. From bellyaches to hemorrhoids, those darn gut discomforts will keep cropping up and get louder and more uncomfortable. You might as well introduce yourself!

One of the ways that we repress uncomfortable feelings and gut sensation is by holding or restricting our breath or by taking shallow breaths (think about the last time something upsetting happened and someone near to us suggested that we "take a deep breath" to relieve some of the pressure.) When we restrict our breath, the gut tightens and the discomfort continues.

Breath is an excellent approach to reconnecting with a disconnected (abandoned) part of ourselves. It has been said that the breath is a bridge between our upper body and our lower body, or our conscious and unconscious minds. Let's initiate the first step towards a functional gut relationship. We can start with a breath to say "hello" to our guts.

Try this: Take a slow, deep breath through your nose, allowing your abdomen to expand. Count to four as you inhale. Now, hold your breath for two counts. Say hello! Now, let the air out slowly, again for four counts, through the nose or mouth.

The relationship begins!

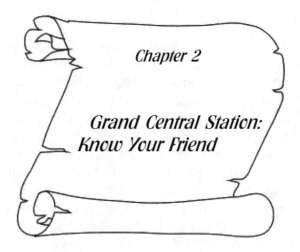

Chapter 2

Grand Central Station:
Know Your Friend

We wear our attitudes in our bodies.

—Patti Davis

 I like to call myself your "Grand Central Station" because of everything I am and everything I do. I am your "receiving" station. I am your "processing" station. I am your "nutrient distribution" station. And finally, I am your "waste elimination" plant. I am changed and altered by each and every thought, emotion, and food you ingest.

If I'm feeling good and working properly, I can receive and process what you "take in," absorb what is life-giving, and eliminate what no longer serves us. But if there is even one glitch in my system, watch out! When I'm miserable, I can make YOU miserable—physically and emotionally.

—Your Gut

Your Personal Plumbing

Once you eat your stir-fried veggies, fruit, or Twinkies, the wisdom of your digestive system goes through quite an amazing process to nourish you. A series of blood vessels and veins wrapped around your stomach, small intestines, and colon absorb vitamins and other nutrients. Most of these nutrients are transferred to your liver, where they are broken down further and then stored, filtered, and distributed via your bloodstream to the rest of your body. While all this is happening, your blood collects waste and eliminates it through your colon, liver, kidney, skin, and lungs.

Each of your digestive organs has an important role in the processing of the foods you eat. But in addition to the physical role these organs play, each organ also has a corresponding psychological role.

As stated in the previous chapter, emotional and psychological responses often go hand in hand with physical responses. Taoist sages as well as various respected body/mind therapists, philosophers, and scientists state that our bodies and minds are so interrelated that it is almost impossible to speak of the body and mind as being separate. Distress or well-being within us will most assuredly influence another. "Thoughts are just one part of our body's [gut's] wisdom. A thought held long enough and repeated enough becomes a belief. The belief then becomes biology," says Dr. Christiane Northrup in her book, *Women's Bodies, Women's Wisdom*. So, while you're reading about the physical functions of each of your organs, take note of the psychological associations. Assimilating this information is just another step towards awareness of the workings of your gut's wisdom.

Eating With Your Head

The table is set, and dinner is served. You smell the food; your mouth begins to water. As you are preparing for your first bite, are you feeling calm and at peace? Are you thinking good thoughts? If so, you are already secreting digestive enzymes (mouth and stomach). A good trip is being prepared for your food's journey of digestion, absorption, and elimination.

If you are depressed, stressed, or anxious before your pearly whites meet your meal, your digestive process is altered often due to either too little digestive enzyme production or too much. Your brain directs signals to your nervous system that, in turn, triggers a cascade of responses along your digestive and elimination system to support or hinder proper digestion.

Mouth

Digestion begins here. Food is chewed, or *masticated*, and mixed with saliva, which contains the enzyme *ptyalin*. Ptyalin begins the digestive process by breaking down starches. (Chew a piece of bread at least 20 times and notice how the flavor changes. It tastes slightly sweet. This is your digestive process breaking the starch down to an easily digestible sugar).

Saliva also contains antibodies that attack bacteria, viruses, and toxins that may have come along for the ride. Chewing your food slowly and thoroughly assists in better digestion and absorption. Chewing thoroughly and moistening your food with saliva allow digestive juices throughout your system to come in full contact with all parts of the food, lessening the chances of gas and other digestive and eliminative imbalances.

**Psychological
Associations:** How do you take in new ideas? Do you take in your nourishment mindfully—physically through your food choices and emotionally through good choices of friends and partners? How do you allow yourself to be nourished? Are you expressing yourself in a way that nourishes and feeds the self and others?

Gut's Wisdom: If imbalances occur, your gut will speak to you with bloat, gas, and undigested food in the bowel movements. You could be overeating and be undernourished. If you are feeling depleted physically and emotionally, it could be due to incomplete digestion and lack of proper nutrient absorption.

Stomach

The stomach is the primary organ for storing and digesting food. When your meal reaches your stomach, nerve impulses alert the central nervous system, which then sends impulses back to your gastric glands to secrete more digestive enzymes. Your emotional status can alter the efficiency of this process (for example, depression or sadness can slow digestion). The stomach is lined with a mucus membrane that protects the stomach tissue from being eaten away by strong stomach acid (hydrochloric acid). The stomach also secretes *prostaglandins*, chemical messengers that are constantly replacing and repairing the stomach lining. The wrong foods, alcohol, smoking, and stress can damage the stomach's protective mucus membrane, creating or exacerbating ulcers. Hydrochloric acid gives your chewed food an acid bath in order to kill any harmful organisms that may infect the rest of your digestive and eliminative tract. It breaks down the proteins (steak, eggs, tofu, fish, beans) in the foods you have chosen into absorbable amino acids. This partially digested food is turned into a liquid called *chyme* and continues its journey into your small intestine. Note: Drinking fluids (including water) with your meals dilutes the digestive process, thereby contributing to gut distress.

**Psychological
Associations:** The stomach symbolizes our ability to "digest" emotional, mental, and spiritual "foods" (thoughts, information, sensations, feelings). Taoists call the stomach the "sea" of nourishment. Do you eat food as a replacement for love and comfort? Do you take in "nourishment" that

enhances your body, mind, and spirit? Are you able to "digest" and take in life experiences easily and utilize them to benefit and enrich yourself? If you are having a difficult time accepting (digesting) an unpalatable or overwhelming experience—something that is "difficult to stomach" or "eats at you"—this can set up a conflict. Your gut may speak to you.

Gut's Wisdom: If imbalances occur, your gut will "speak" to you with indigestion, gastritis, belching, constipation, vomiting, ulcers, or heartburn.

Small Intestine

The small intestine is a 25-foot-long coil of tubing in charge of completing the digestion and absorption of your foods and separating the pure from the toxic. After the food is broken down in the stomach, a valve opens up and the chyme (your partially digested food) is released into the uppermost part of the small intestine, called the duodenum. As it passes into the duodenum, enzymes from the pancreas are released to further break down fats, proteins, and carbohydrates. The pancreatic juices are alkaline, which neutralize acidic stomach acids, thereby protecting the small intestinal lining. Hormones in your blood stimulate the gall bladder to release bile to break down fats. This entire process makes the nutrients from our foods into usable and absorbable forms.

The small intestine is where absorption—one of the most vital functions of the digestive system—occurs. If you aren't absorbing nutrients efficiently, your health is jeopardized. The small intestine takes the usable nutrients from your food and sends them into the bloodstream via the *villi*—five million fingerlike projections. These villi line the small intestine and contain blood and lymph capillaries. The nutrients are delivered via the blood capillaries to your liver for further filtering before being released to your system. Fats are transformed from the villi into the lymphatic system for distribution. The villi also protect by blocking the absorption of foreign substances that are not useful to the body. An overuse of certain medications, alcohol, poorly digested food, and stress can destroy the small intestine's protective barrier, allowing toxic substances to seep into the bloodstream. This often contributes to body-wide symptoms labeled as leaky-gut syndrome.

Of the nutrients you need to survive, 90 percent or more are absorbed from the small intestine, feeding your entire body. All that isn't absorbed gets passed on to the large intestine for elimination.

Psychological
Associations: The small intestine's job is assimilating, absorbing, and separating. Taoists label the small intestine as the "controller for the transformation of matter." The small intestine is in charge of separating the "pure" from the "impure"—not only within food, but also from thoughts and emotions.

Just as too much unassimilated food clogs the intestines and weighs down the body, so too will unassimilated thoughts and feelings burden the spirit. These unassimilated thoughts and feelings can make you feel stressed out, mentally and emotionally "stuffed," defensive, uncomfortable, and/or scattered. Do you process and utilize the information, ideas, and feelings that are present in your life, or do you hold on, clogging your gut and mind? Are you able to discern what is "toxic" in your life and receive what is life-enhancing and nourishing?

Gut's Wisdom: If imbalances occur, your gut will "speak" with bloat (which often "armors" the belly against feelings too difficult to absorb), allergies, candida, elimination problems such as constipation or diarrhea, leaky-gut syndrome, malabsorption, or immune system challenges.

Pancreas

The pancreas has two main jobs: the production of digestive enzymes and the production of insulin. As food passes from the stomach to the duodenum (the upper portion of the small intestine), the pancreas secretes bicarbonates that reduce the acidity of the chyme in order to prevent irritation of the intestinal tissues. The pancreas manufactures and secretes enzymes such as lipase, amylase, and protease, which assist in breaking down fats, carbohydrates, and proteins. The pancreas produces insulin, a hormone that regulates blood sugar levels within the body. The more coffee, sugar, and refined flour products we ingest, the harder the pancreas has to work. If the pancreas becomes imbalanced, hypoglycemia and diabetes may develop.

Psychological

Associations: Are you able to find and appreciate the "sweetness of life?" Or are you all work and no play?

Gut's Wisdom: If imbalances occur, you may experience hypoglycemia, diabetes, cravings for sweets, loose stools, bloating, headaches, nausea, fatigue, irritability, insomnia, anxiety, or depression.

Immune Protectors

Research indicates that a majority of the immune system is located within the digestive tract. Your digestive tract is especially rich in lymphatic tissue, which is a major part of your immune system. As much as 70 percent of Gut Associated Lymph Tissue (GALT) is located in the lining of your digestive tract and in the intestinal mucosa.

In portions of your small intestine, there are nodules of lymph tissue called Peyers patches that contain lymphocytes whose purpose is to attach to any unsavory bacteria that has managed to get into your gut. These lymphocytes alert other protective cells to act to rid the gut of the bacteria.

Psychological

Associations: The major job of the immune system is to recognize any foreign substances and thereby come to the rescue in order to prevent these substances from doing us harm. This represents the ability to discern and to defend ourselves against attack and invasion. Do you allow others' thoughts and actions to offend or "infect" you, creating a defensive biochemistry? Do you feel powerless? Are you harboring feelings of guilt, criticism, self-hatred, or resentment against yourself or another? Are you out of touch with your inner strengths and feelings? If so, the result can be throwing your system out of balance.

Gut's Wisdom: A weakened immune system increases susceptibility to virtually every type of illness. Some common signs include listlessness, fatigue, allergic reactions, repeated infections, inflammation, candida, and vaginal yeast infections. A variety of many disorders, such as lupus, rheumatoid arthritis, AIDS, and cancer, have been linked to compromised immune system activity.

Secretory IgA (S(IgA))

S(IgA) is an antibody that is also found in the intestinal mucosa. It is in the saliva as well as throughout the entire digestive and eliminative tract. S(IgA) molecules are on constant alert to defend against foreign invaders (bacteria, antigens, viruses, and parasites). What you eat, how well you digest and eliminate, and—most significantly—your emotional health have impact on the fortitude of the S(IgA) antibodies.

Psychological Associations: The major job of the immune system is to recognize any foreign substances and thereby come to the rescue in order to prevent these substances from doing us harm. This represents the ability to discern and to defend ourselves against attack and invasion. Do you allow others' thoughts and actions to offend or "infect" you, creating a defensive biochemistry? Do you feel powerless? Are you harboring feelings of guilt, criticism, self-hatred, or resentment against yourself or another? Are you out of touch with your inner strengths and feelings? If so, the result can be throwing your system out of balance.

Gut's Wisdom: A weakened immune system increases susceptibility to virtually every type of illness. Some common signs include listlessness, fatigue, allergic reactions, repeated infections, inflammation, candida, and vaginal yeast infections. A variety of many disorders, such as lupus, rheumatoid arthritis, AIDS, and cancer, have been linked to compromised immune system activity.

Appendix

After the nutrients have been extracted from your meal, the chyme passes through a valve called the ileo-cecal valve into the large intestine. Here, your chyme meets up with your appendix.

The appendix is a small sac (1 to 6 inches) that hangs off the beginning of your large intestine. Some researchers and doctors believe that the appendix is obsolete or some mystery appendage; some other doctors believe otherwise. Dr. Norman Walker, the author of *Colon Health,* has written that its job is to secrete a germicidal mucus to kill off toxins that have entered the large intestine. Some recent research has suggested that the appendix contains lymphatic tissue and may be an important part of our immune system's function for destroying infectious bacteria.

Psychological
Associations: The major job of the immune system is to recognize any foreign substances and thereby come to the rescue in order to prevent these substances from doing us harm. This represents the ability to discern and to defend ourselves against attack and invasion. Do you allow others' thoughts and actions to offend or "infect" you, creating a defensive biochemistry? Do you feel powerless? Are you harboring feelings of guilt, criticism, self-hatred, or resentment against yourself or another? Are you out of touch with your inner strengths and feelings? If so, the result can be throwing your system out of balance.

Gut's Wisdom: Fever, nausea, pain, constipation, and distress around the navel. There's tenderness to the right of the navel and below, which is there the appendix is situated.

Large Intestine

Also known as the colon or the bowel, the large intestine is the last 5 feet of your gastrointestinal tract. The main function of the large intestine is to act as a holding tank for our waste products. Waste products are held in this region, as water and electrolytes are absorbed into the body. If waste moves through the large intestine too quickly, water is not absorbed, resulting in diarrhea. Conversely, if waste does not move through the large intestine normally, it becomes hard and dry, resulting in difficult-to-pass waste; this is better known as constipation. A small amount of mucus is secreted—and acts as a gentle lubricant to protect the colon's delicate lining from too much acidity and toxins. Water is absorbed as the waste matter moves along towards the rectum and anus for elimination. Approximately two-thirds of the waste matter is composed of water, undigested fibers, and digested food products. The other third is composed of dead cells and living and dead bacteria. Within the large intestine, there is an abundance of intestinal bacteria—up to 500 species—along with a mixture of yeast and fungi, all in a delicate ecological balance. There are "friendly" bacteria, which are health-promoting, neutral bacteria, and "unfriendly" bacteria, which are disease-causing and toxic. Each of these is competing for a place to take up residence and multiply. The "friendly" bacteria synthesize vitamin K (a blood-clotting agent) and manufacture B vitamins. Other bacteria protect the gut from inflammation and infection. "Unfriendly" bacteria are gas- and disease-causing bacteria. A recommended balance is 80 percent "friendly" bacteria and 20 percent "unfriendly" bacteria. Antibiotics, poor food choices, inadequate digestion, and stress can throw off this delicate balance, causing a whole array of gut ailments.

Waste is moved through your colon by rhythmic muscular contractions called *peristalsis*. Fiber supports the process of peristalsis. The bulkier, more fibrous, waste matter can travel faster through the large intestine, because it has been provided with substances with which the colon musculature can work. If the large intestine is not working properly, the muscles of the colon can be come stretched out, or "ballooned," and become lazy or spastic. This can cause absorption of toxins back into our systems and wreak havoc physically and emotionally. A hard-to-believe fact: An unhealthy colon has been reported to "hold" up to *15-plus pounds* of waste material.

Psychological
Associations: The large intestine is the drainage ditch or the gut-brain garbage collector. It is the holding tank for what no longer benefits us. It is a reflection of our overall physical and emotional health. It mirrors our issues around trusting, letting go of the *old* emotions, attitudes, and beliefs, in order to make room for the *new*. Do you hold on to toxic or limiting beliefs, unexpressed or unresolved feelings? Do you feel "stuck," or do you let go with ease?

Gut's wisdom: If imbalances occur, so many things stem from an improperly functioning colon: constipation, irritable bowel syndrome (IBS), diarrhea, fatigue, skin conditions, muscle aches and pains, headaches, depression, allergies—you name it!

Liver

The liver is the largest organ in the body. It is located above the stomach, beneath the right side of the rib cage, under the diaphragm. It is the only organ that can regenerate its damaged tissue. This is especially true when it receives proper nutritional support.

Our liver function is compromised by inadequate diet choices of refined flour and sugar products, alcohol, and coffee, as well as medications, food and environmental chemicals, and stress. The liver does its best to detoxify what it can, but, if it is compromised, it will store the toxins in the liver cells and within the tissues and organs throughout the body. The repercussions can leave you with allergies, chronic fatigue, skin problems, chronic digestive and elimination ailments, an impaired immune system, hormonal imbalances, and mood swings. The Gut Wisdom Cleanse (Chapter 9) will help modify these imbalances.

Basically, the health of your liver is a major determinant of the health of your entire body. The liver has a full-time job of being responsible for more than 500 functions. It metabolizes proteins, fats, and carbohydrates into forms your body can use as fuel; manufactures natural antihistamines; forms and stores red blood cells; makes and breaks down hormones; and is the only organ that can detoxify your blood.

The liver can be likened to a large sieve that filters everything in the blood before it is distributed to feed your body. Blood flows from the intestinal tract to the liver, where it is filtered and where toxins and hormones are neutralized and deactivated, rendering them harmless. Along with detoxifying the intestinal tract, a healthy liver also deactivates heavy metals such as lead, mercury, and aluminum, as well as food additives, pesticides, nicotine, alcohol, and drugs and medications. Nutrients are then excreted via the kidneys and eliminated via bile through the colon.

Bile is manufactured by the liver then secreted into and temporarily stored in the gall bladder. Bile is made of bile salts, cholesterol, lecithin, hormones, and electrolytes. Bile gives the stool its brown color. It helps lubricate the intestines and assists in breaking down fat, as well as supports the absorption of valuable fat-soluble vitamins. Bile carries many of the toxins from the liver into the intestines. Normally, bile is flushed out with the help of fiber. If the diet is high in fat and low in fiber, a high concentration of bile can linger in the intestines. The toxins can be recirculated back into the bloodstream to all body tissues and organs, resulting in a myriad of body ailments caused by autointoxification (self-poisoning). In addition to overtaxing the liver, the toxin-filled bile can become irritating to the intestinal lining as well as a contributing factor to the development of cancer.

Another job of the liver is the production of antihistamines to neutralize allergic responses. If the liver is congested and overworked with more toxins than it can detoxify, histamines will increase, triggering an allergic response from the foods you eat to the environmental pollutants and potential allergens around you.

Hormones, such as testosterone and estrogen, are metabolized by the liver. This process is jeopardized if the liver function is compromised along with a lack of certain vitamin Bs (required by the liver to support the detoxification of estrogen) and an insufficient amount of "friendly" bacteria inhabiting the gut. Improperly metabolized estrogen results in the production of toxic estrogen by-products. If the colon doesn't eliminate these by-products efficiently, PMS, bloating, and excessive moodiness, as well as other hormonal-related ailments, may arise.

The liver must also metabolize certain hormones such as adrenaline and cortisol—the stress-related, fight-or-flight hormones. These can poison our bodies, especially if we are on a regular diet of worry, frustration, and anger. Hormones can be stored for *up to a year* in the liver, adding to emotional imbalances, such as chronic anger and depression. This, in turn, suppresses the immune system. It's not surprising then that Webster's dictionary defines "liverish" as displaying a sour disposition, peevish or cross, or that the word *melancholy* came from the Greek *melano* (black) and *chole* (bile). Traditional Chinese medicine calls this liverish state "liver stagnation." Western medicine calls this "sluggish liver." Whatever you call it, excess hormones and toxins not eliminated by a poorly functioning liver give an already stressed-out person a truly peevish personality.

The liver produces natural antihistamines. If the liver is impaired to the point of not performing its important function(s), the body and gut may react negatively to various foods and environmental conditions. These conditions include allergies, hay fever, digestive and eliminative challenges, headaches, skin conditions, depression, irritability, and fatigue.

Waste filtered from the blood by the liver is carried through the intestinal tract and eliminated. If this process isn't working properly (if we don't have daily bowel movements), the wastes are reabsorbed through the colon wall, recycled through our body, and delivered right back to the liver—again.

Whew! Almost every bodily function depends on the liver. This is a very overworked organ.

Psychological
Associations: According to Taoists, the liver has the function of a CEO whose specialty is strategic planning. A lack of planning or follow-through results in frustration. Anger is the emotion connected with the liver. When there is an obstruction of

feelings and bottled-up frustration, this may result in anger, often alternating with depression. Do you experience anger, mood swings, depression, a negative outlook, and indecision?

Gut's Wisdom: If imbalances occur, you may experience sluggish bowels, fatigue, nausea, dizziness, yellowish skin or itching, intolerance of fatty and oily foods, gas, bloat, liver spots, PMS, food allergies, hemorrhoids, inability to lose weight, depression, melancholy, anger, and temper.

Gall Bladder

The gall bladder is a sack attached to the underside of your liver. Its job is to store and concentrate bile produced by the liver. As you eat, your gall bladder releases bile via a common duct that connects the liver, gall bladder, and the pancreas into the duodenum (upper section of the small intestine). Bile neutralizes stomach acids, thereby protecting the delicate intestinal lining from irritation. Bile is an important component of the digestion of fats and fat-soluble vitamins. Bile also assists in the peristalsis and helps prevent fermentation in the gut. Internally produced and environmental toxins are eliminated via the bile that has been filtered through the liver. The bile is what gives color to your daily bowel movement. Absence of bile secretion results in light, clay-colored stool. Bile is reabsorbed into the bloodstream when the gall bladder bile duct becomes blocked, such as due to gall stones (when cholesterol and bile pigments crystallize together) or infection (for example, hepatitis: a yellowish hue, known as jaundice, will show up in the whites of your eyes and skin).

Psychological Associations: According to ancient Chinese philosophers, the gall bladder is called "the decision maker." The gallbladder (and liver) is also affected by anger, frustration, and repressed bitterness or resentment. Do you "go with the flow" and trust, or do you attempt to control? Do you have pent-up anger and resentment? Gallstones can indicate hard thoughts and bitterness. Controlling behavior and indecision are psychological earmarks of an imbalance.

Gut's Wisdom: If there is an imbalance you may experience pain under right ribs, gall stones, nausea, vomiting, a bitter taste in the mouth, yellow color in the whites of eyes and skin, "temple" headaches, stiffness and pain in the shoulder, chronic gas, belching, bloating, bowel sluggishness, and pale/light-colored stools.

Diaphragm and Solar Plexus

The diaphragm is a muscular plate positioned below the lungs and above the stomach, liver, and solar plexus. It is our main respiratory muscle that is essential for the breathing process. With each deep inhalation, it gently massages and stimulates the abdominal organs, enhancing the intestine's peristaltic action. With each exhalation, it assists toxins out of the lungs.

The diaphragm allows us to breathe deeply and let go of tension and stress. A tight/tense diaphragm is experienced as a restricted or shallow breath, creating a block to our emotions—and it is very susceptible to emotional stress. As we feel frustration, anger, or loss of control, the flight-or-flight reflex tightens the abdominal muscles. There is minimal room for our diaphragm to go through its full range of motion. As the breath remains restricted, the diaphragm tightens, and digestion and elimination suffer due to a lack of stimulation. The diaphragm has a direct effect on the solar plexus.

The solar plexus is a collection of nerves just below the diaphragm. It is the largest autonomic nerve center in the abdominal cavity. It affects the adrenal glands, which are responsible for the regulation and distribution of metabolic energy within the body. It also affects the digestive system—the stomach, liver, and gall bladder—which assists the body in its assimilation of nutrients.

The solar plexus is often labeled "the seat of the emotions." This is where we experience those "butterfly" sensations when we are nervous and where we receive our "gut feelings," which intuitively guide us. It is the core of our inner knowing and personal power. It is our gut wisdom's central home.

Psychological Associations: The solar plexus is a central point of our inner knowing as well as a reflection of all our fears, especially the fear of losing control. There may be an obsession about controlling others or self. It is associated with the expression of your will (your personal power).

Do you feel and express your truth? Or are you overly influenced by outside influences and feel like a victim? As you use your personal power, do you respect others or do you attempt to bully them? Diaphragm tension occurs as one represses and ignores gut feelings. According to Wilhelm Reich, a pioneer in body/mind therapy, a tightened diaphragm (which blocks the solar plexus) correlates with a psychological armoring. As it armors or blocks unexpressed anger and frustrations, it can also block feelings of joy, sexuality, and honest expressions of emotion.

Gut's Wisdom: When this area is blocked, the gut speaks with digestive and elimination ailments, indigestion, IBS, constipation, ulcers, adrenal exhaustion, menstrual ailments, eating disorders, and a pot belly.

"One of the most important indicators of what actions to take with respect to our health is the presence of lack of ease in the pit of your stomach or 'gut brain' when thoughtfully reflecting on your options."

—Mark Percival, *The Mind Body Connection*

The Delicate Balance

So you see what a complex and beautiful thing the digestive and elimination system—your gut—really is. But as are many complex and beautiful things, the gut is also sensitive. If you do not respect your gut, and if the delicate balance in the system is disturbed, it can trigger a host of chemical and systemic reactions that can result in a series of gut and body-wide ailments. Then things can get really serious.

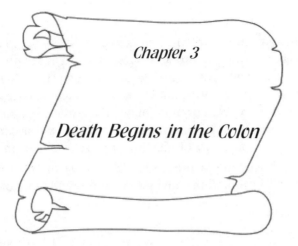

Chapter 3

Death Begins in the Colon

The very best diets can be no better than the very worst, if the sewage system of the colon is clogged with a collection of waste and corruption.

—Norman Walker, D.C., Ph.D.

I know this sounds pretty dramatic, but I have major jobs to attend to. If I am not getting sufficient attention, I will tenaciously make myself heard any way I can in any part of your body. Remember: I feed every cell within you. If your skin is broken out, or your muscles ache or your thinking is fuzzy, look to me! I just may have a finger—or a villi—in it!

The more you learn about me and the things I need, the more steps you take to keep me healthy, the happier we both will be.

—Your Gut

I was raised hearing my father say "death begins in the colon"—over and over again. As a kid, I hated it. It was negative and downright scary. For my father, however, it turned out to be tragically correct. And as my years as a colon therapist unfolded, I saw over and over again how an unhealthy colon could lead to digestive and intestinal dysfunction and prolonged illness, as well as our everyday physical and emotional ailments.

Our digestive and elimination system's job is to convert the foods we eat into energy for our body, then package up what's left over and easily send it out of our body. Many of our food selections don't support that job. Also, when we take in "food for thought" that is stressed-filled and not nourishing, our natural healthy gut function is additionally affected.

Disease begins in the colon when the digestive and elimination system is not in top-notch working order. This is particularly true if the colon has become sluggish, constipated, and weak. A sluggish *dysfunctional* colon cannot properly eliminate wastes and toxins. Medical science now acknowledges that up to 85 percent or more of all adult Americans suffer some sort of intestinal imbalance. It's inevitable that toxins will accumulate in the colon resulting in some sort of ailment—the gut's voice—in the body.

So what constitutes a functional (healthy) or dysfunctional (unhealthy) colon? Let me introduce you to the inhabitants of your colon.

Bacteria

An abundance of "friendly" and "unfriendly" (harmful) bacteria inhabits the gut. The goal of a healthy gut is to house more friendly bacteria than unfriendly.

The gut houses more bacteria than your body has cells. There are up to 500 different species of bacteria within the gastrointestinal (GI) tract. The most important species is lactobacillus acidophilus in the small intestine (which is killed with the use of antibiotics and affected by stress). Its job is to keep the digestive track healthy and functioning efficiently. It helps promote nutrient absorption and healthy digestion, as well as assists another valuable bacteria, bifidobacterium, which is found in your large intestine. These "friendly" bacteria are the defenders, detoxifiers, and protectors against viruses and unfriendly bacteria invading your system. Ideally, your gut should contain approximately 80 percent "friendly" bacteria to 20 percent "unfriendly" bacteria.

Dybosis

Bacteria balance plays a major role in our ability to prevent and fight infections and disease. It is our first line of protection in our immune system's defense. When the unfriendly bacteria take charge of the gut's delicate environment, a state called *dybosis* occurs. Dybosis means "not living together in mutual harmony." When this disruption is present, the gut is left open to the overgrowth of yeast, fungi, parasites, and potentially harmful (toxic) strains of bacteria.

Repercussions of Dybosis: Certain bacteria in the colon, such as members of the clostridium family (associated with high fat and meat eaters), are associated with intestinal toxicity. These bacteria, when left to live in an imbalanced bacteria environment, have the ability to metabolize unabsorbed nutrients or food by-products such as bile acids, fatty acids, or cholesterol and convert them into toxic substances such as carcinogens. (Bile acids are believed to be one of the risk factors for colon cancer. If they remain too long in the gut, they can be converted by colonic bacteria into carcinogens.)

■ ■ ■ ■ ■ ■ ■ ■ ■

How the Unfriendly Bacteria
Take Charge of the Gut's Environment

Bacterial balance is disrupted by emotional stress, illness, antibiotics, steroid drugs, medications, chemotherapy and radiation, birth control pills, slow bowel transit time, environmental chemicals, and poor food choices, such as sugar, fast foods high in fat, meat diets, and/or alcohol indulgence.

■ ■ ■

When friendly bacteria are in charge in your GI tract:

▷ The immune system is strong.

▷ There is little putrefaction in the gut. Gas is minimized, and waste moves out easily and quickly.

▷ The gut is protected from disease-causing opportunistic microorganisms such as yeast, fungus (candida albicans), E-coli, H-pylori, and salmonella.

▷ Abdominal tenderness, inflammation, and constipation are lessened.

▷ Vaginal infections are kept to a minimum.

▷ Resistance to food poisoning is increased.

▷ Nutrient production, digestion, and absorption are increased.

▷ Toxins are neutralized.

Critters and Creepy Crawlies

The gut can also be home to all kinds of organisms that most of us don't want to think about but that can affect the health of our guts, and thus, the health of our entire systems.

Candida

Candida is a fungus that lives quietly inside all of us in small amounts, unless our gut's friendly bacteria gets thrown out of balance and the immune system is compromised. Candida is associated with a dybosis process known as fermentation. Individuals with fermentation dybosis have inadequate digestion of carbohydrates (that is, grains, sugar, fruit, beer, and wine). The gut speaks with excessive gas, bloat, diarrhea, constipation, and fatigue, as well as a host of other body-wide symptoms (See "Candida Albicans" in Chapter 10).

Parasites

Just the *idea* of parasites in our systems makes most of us shiver. Yet we are used as residences by more than 130 species of parasites. If dybosis is present and our digestion is dysfunctional, parasites can make themselves at home and create toxic by-products that contribute to gut inflammation, irritation, and gut toxicity. More than you realize, many of us are affected by one or more of these gut invaders. (See "Parasites" in Chapter 10.)

Putrefaction

This, essentially, is when food is rotting inside you—not a pretty thought. This dybosis occurs when food is not properly digested or eliminated. Slow bowel transit time, poorly combined foods, digestive enzyme deficiency, lack of fiber, too much fat, excess animal protein, sugar, stress, and eating when not relaxed are all contributors to putrefaction in your gut.

If the bowels are "sluggish," the waste and toxic by-products from the food we eat build up to such an extent that they become putrefied (I dislike the sound of that, but that's the process). In short, if the "garbage" doesn't get taken out, it begins to rot. The putrefaction builds up and becomes a breeding ground for colonies of undesirable toxin-producing, disease-causing bacteria that can get absorbed into our bloodstream.

Many cancer researchers agree that cancer can be caused by exposure or contact with cancer-causing chemicals known as carcinogens. In a sluggish bowel, harmless bile that comes in contact with putrefactive bacteria can actually be *converted* into dangerous carcinogens.

Autointoxication: What Doesn't Get Eliminated Gets Recirculated

In a perfect world and a functional gut, the colon completes the digestive process. It absorbs minerals, nutrients, and excess water from the digested residue of the food we've eaten and discharges toxins and waste materials from the body. When the colon is clean and healthy, we experience a feeling of well-being. When it is congested with fermenting, putrefying gases, stagnant wastes and toxins can recirculate into the system and pollute our inner environment: *What is not eliminated is recirculated.* This gut dysfunction is labeled autointoxication (literally, self-poisoning). Autointoxication occurs when we ingest and/or create more waste than we can eliminate through all our body's eliminative channels (bowels, kidneys, lungs, skin, lymphatic system).

Here's what happens: Once the first layer of mucoid fecal matter forms on the walls of the colon, further layers develop more easily as the peristaltic action becomes slower and slower. The muscular wall of the intestines and colon can atrophy just as other muscles can, which makes it harder for them to contract and relax and pass their contents. Here is the beginning of a myriad of digestive and eliminative problems, such as constipation, diarrhea (the body's attempt to clean itself out), gas, cramping, IBS, and more. Weakened bowel muscles can then contribute to the formation of *diverticuli*, which are little pouches that balloon out from the colon muscle wall in which fecal material collects and festers toxic bacteria festers. These pouches can actually rupture, spilling dangerous, life-threatening toxins into the gut and bloodstream.

The colon's condition does not have to get to such a serious state before toxins within the colon can make their way into the blood and lymphatic system through the intestinal wall and deposit themselves in the tissues and organs of our body. The example I often give is living in a house in which the gas from the stove is left on, but the windows are cracked. The effects of the poisons are slow but far-reaching.

Also, the bacteria within the gut interact with the stagnant waste, and toxic chemicals and gases are created. These toxins can cause damage to the mucosal lining, resulting in increased intestinal permeability, a condition known as leaky-gut syndrome. Toxins, bacteria, viruses, and parasites, now without boundaries, are able to spread throughout the body via the bloodstream.

These toxins that get absorbed into our bodies are often sent to the liver. The liver is the first line of defense against toxins entering the blood. If your liver is not working optimally—because of overindulgence in food, alcohol, medications, and stress—your sensitivity to toxins increases. If the toxins back up into your system, your cells may hold extra water to dilute them and you become bloated; excess weight and cellulite occur. You feel nauseas if they reach the stomach and foul-breathed if they reach the lungs. Muscles ache or become inflamed. Nerve fibers become irritated, leaving you easily agitated. Mental fog and headaches are chronic conditions. If the toxins back up to the skin—another organ of elimination—it becomes sallow and blemished, and often rashes, discolorations, and wrinkles can occur. And if the toxins back up into the glands, you feel tired and often catch the latest "bug" that's going around. You lack spark and sex drive and can look old beyond your years.

Unfortunately, we usually treat the symptoms resulting from the toxic overload, rather than the cause of these symptoms. Even if one succeeds in suppressing a symptom with medications, the toxic flow from the bowel will simply find another area through which it can detoxify, thereby overworking, stressing, and weakening other organs. This is the gut's way of attempting to preserve our health. It wants to rid us of these toxins.

According to the Royal Society of Medicine in Great Britain article "Death Begins in the Colon," almost every known chronic disease is due directly or indirectly to the influence of more than 36 bacterial poisons that are absorbed from the intestines into our blood streams. In the book *Tissue Cleansing Through Bowel Management*, Dr. Bernard Jensen states, "intestinal toxins must be eliminated before any treatment method—no matter how sophisticated—can overcome disease." *A gut cleanse is mandatory!* (See Chapter 9.)

Look at it this way: If our city's sewer system backed up into our water system, the sanitation department would immediately fix the problem before the health of city citizens was jeopardized. Our colon is our *personal sewer system*; it needs care and repair to maintain our personal health.

To no other single cause is it possible to attribute one-tenth as many various and widely diverse disorders. A dysfunctionally operating, clogged, irritated, and weak colon may be looked upon as a veritable Pandora's box, out of which spring misery and suffering—emotional and mental as well as physical.

Exposed: Dysfunctions of the Colon

Your colon is a muscle that, when neglected with years of stress, bad eating, and neglectful behaviors, can prolapse, stretch, spasm, balloon, or even become cancerous.

Normal

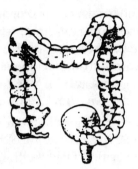

This is the ideal colon (large intestine): no kinks and no stretched, ballooned, or irritated areas. Lucky guy!

■ ■ ■ ■ ■ ■ ⌐ ■ ■

Prolapsus

A sagging (prolapsed) colon. Most often, this sagging is found in the transverse section of the intestine, usually due to the weight of waste material accumulated there. Chronic constipation and poor digestion are culprits. The prolapsed section of the intestine may also press on the bladder, uterus, or prostate, contributing to other problems.

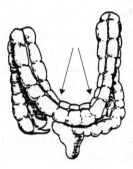

■ ■ ■ ■ ■ ■ ■ ■ ■

Diverticulosis

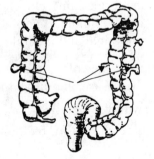

When waste is constipated and dehydrated, it is more difficult to push through the colon. Pressure builds up and causes a "blowout"—a pocket in the intestinal wall. Waste can get trapped in these ruptures or small herniations (diverticula). As this progresses, inflammation, cramping, and fevers may occur—a condition called diverticulitis.

Ballooning

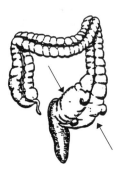

Ballooning often occurs in the sigmoid portion of the large intestine. Chronic constipation can cause a severe stretching of the muscles of the intestines, allowing copious amounts of waste to linger. A full, ballooned lower bowel is both uncomfortable and distressing, and it can also put pressure on the prostate and left ovary and can contribute to hemorrhoids.

■　■　■　■　■　■　■　■　■　■

Irritable Bowel Syndrome

Irritable bowel syndrome, an umbrella name given to a group of bowel symptoms: colitis, inflammation, tenderness, abdominal muscle spasms and cramping, and chronic diarrhea and constipation that dance back and forth. Besides the feeling that your life is being controlled by your bowels, you may also experience lower backaches from the erratic spasms of your colon.

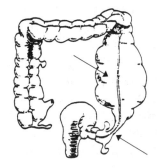

■　■　■　■　■　■　■　■　■　■

Colon Cancer

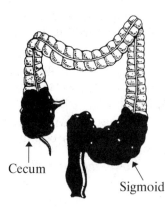

Cecum

Sigmoid

Eighty percent of bowel cancers affect these two areas: the cecum (beginning part of the ascending colon) and the last portion of the colon, known as the sigmoid. These are the areas that tend to accumulate waste matter that becomes the perfect breeding ground for harmful, unfriendly, putrefying bacteria within the gut.

The toxic, dysfunctional gut affects the entire body as it attempts to rid itself of toxins via all the eliminative organs (lungs, kidneys, skin, and bowels). But when some of what should have been eliminated is recirculated, the following symptoms can arise:

- Colitis.
- Skin problems (acne, eczema, itching).
- Hemorrhoids.
- Fatigue.
- Nausea.
- Weakened immune system.
- Liver problems.
- Cancer.
- Foul gas.
- Muscular aches and pains.
- Indigestion.
- PMS.
- Gall stones.
- Irritable Bowel Syndrome (IBS).
- Appendicitis.
- Allergies.
- Distended abdomen.
- "-itis" inflammatory conditions (arthritis, sinusitis, diverticulitis).
- Sleep disturbances.
- Bad breath.
- Body odor.
- Diarrhea.
- Headaches/migraines.
- Indecision.
- Mental fog.
- Depression.
- Weight gain.
- Melancholy.
- Irritability.
- Hypertension (high blood pressure).
- Frequent illness.
- Constipation.

You see that the healthy functioning of your gut is vital to the health of your entire body. Through these symptoms, the gut's wisdom attempts to get our attention.

A Functional Bowel Movement

Knowing and not doing is equal to not knowing.

—Chinese proverb

Emperors in China had their waste matter examined to check their health status. Parents are concerned with their children's bowel movements. Dog owners often check their pets' dropping for worms, loose stools, or "good ones" to determine their best friends' health. However, as adults, we don't even want to think about what goes into the toilet, let alone look at it!

The value of understanding, interpreting, or knowing what is being deposited in the toilet can give you insight to what is happening internally in your digestive and elimination systems. By taking a peek, you can receive guidance on what new choices you can make for your gut's health.

If you are passing round balls or irregular shaped stool, this can point to a lack of fiber, water, and friendly bacteria. Mucus in the stools may indicate an irritated colon, such as colitis. A diet with mucus-producing foods, such as cheese, milk, or foods you may be allergic or sensitive to can also create mucus. A microorganism, such as candida, can irritate the gut, causing excessive mucus. Foul-smelling and sink-to-the-bottom-of-the-toilet stools may indicate poor food digestion or insufficient fiber, water, and/ or unfriendly bacteria. Greasy or oily stools, which need extra Charmin to wipe off, can be an indication that fats are not being properly digested. Difficult, incomplete, painful, or you-have-time-to-read-a-chapter-of-this-book stools can mean that more water, fiber, and/or friendly bacteria are in order. Blood showing up in the stool can be a hemorrhoid that has ruptured or a more serious health problem (see your doctor!). A normal bowel movement should be a healthy, *easy* discharge of waste matter, not an event that causes pain and distress.

■ ■ ■ ■ ■ ■ ■ ■ ■

Characteristics of a Functional Bowel Movement

- Easy and effortless to pass. No strain, grunts, and moans. No need or time to read another chapter of *Gut Wisdom*. You are *letting go* of what no longer serves you.
- "Floaters" instead of sinking stools indicate you're ingesting enough fiber and water. You're digesting your food efficiently.
- 2 inches in width and 6 inches in length is the optimum goal.
- Fawn-colored (medium brown) is ideal, unless you are ingesting lots of green veggies (you may see a greenish hue) or if you eat a lot of protein (a very dark brown).
- Minimum to no odor when the deed is done.
- An easy wipe experience.
- Feeling empty and complete.

■ ■ ■

Most likely, if you are reading this book you have not achieved the perfect functional bowel movement yet. Chances are you may not be listening to the messages your gut has been sending you. By ignoring the message, you're killing the messenger: your gut's wisdom.

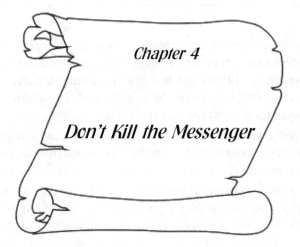

Chapter 4

Don't Kill the Messenger

We will begin to get well when we are tired of being sick.

—Lao Tzu

I've been doing my best to get your attention—cramps, constipation, bloat, irritation, diarrhea, backaches. I've annoyed you, I've pained you, I've dazed and confused you, yet you still try to drown me out with pills and food and frantic activity.

Look, unlike the brain in your head, I can't play emotional, self-defeating games. I can't rationalize, lie, project, attack, or blame. I cannot convince myself of anything or talk myself out of anything. I cannot hide the truth. I'm pure reaction, pure sensation. I'm *you* at your most guileless, your most authentic. I remind you to eat better food and get more rest, I inform you who and what to be afraid of, I alert you to the fact that there are undigested traumas, unhealed emotional experiences, old hurts that need redressing.

What do I have to do to get you to listen?

—Your Gut

I remember years ago when I was in denial about the warning signals in my life. I was driving my favorite Toyota Celica and a red light appeared on the panel next to *oil*. "Oh, how annoying. I'll attend to it later," I thought, while placing a recently acquired business card over the light.

Weeks later, driving through town, I heard a noise. It sounded as if it was coming from underneath my hood. What an inconvenience! I didn't like the noise, nor did I like the hassle of stopping and checking it out; I had things to do, errands to run. So I increased the volume of my eight-track Boz Skags tape to drown out the noise.

A few days after that, as I was driving down the expressway, smoke began to pour out from underneath the hood—smoke so intense I could no longer see ahead of me.

And then the car stopped dead.

It was only when I got stranded on the highway that I realized how big a problem I really had. It was only then that I became *aware*.

Awareness, Awareness, Awareness

When individuals come to see me at my center or workshops, they usually arrive in some sort of gut distress. I greet them with compassion and enthusiasm, for now they have the opportunity to reconnect with a disconnected part of self. Their guts have gotten their attention. Their guts have triggered a desire for *awareness.*

Awareness is the ability to acknowledge and honor what is being messengered to you via your symptoms. If I had a magic wand and could take away all my clients' gut aches and pains, chances are they'd keep doing all those things that gave them unhealthy guts in the first place! Every painful symptom in your belly is your gut's wisdom—a warning that something needs attending to. When we dismiss our cars' warning lights, we have many happy and prosperous mechanics. Likewise, with the regular avoidance of our guts' guidance and warning voice, we have happy and prosperous pharmaceutical companies and doctors.

Many of us have gotten *disconnected* as our fast-paced lifestyles have directed us towards fast foods and superficial remedies, leading us away from what truly nourishes us and supports good health. We have lost what we authentically *feel*, *need*, and *want.* We have shut or repressed our grief, our tears, our wants, our needs, our guidance. We have become talking heads, and we avoid listening to the wisdom of our feelings and emotions contained within our gut.

"Emotions are produced by glandular and visceral reactions to our environment. Therefore our feelings and emotions can help us be aware and tune into the stressors in our life. They give us guidance about what we desire, need, lack or what is still unhealed," says Dr. Candace Pert in her book, *Molecules of Emotion*.

To heal, we must be aware of what we are feeding ourselves, physically, emotionally, and mentally. Our gut and body need proper food and nutrients to function optimally. Our gut works best when being fed with positive, nourishing thoughts. We need to allow our emotions to flow, to be felt, to be expressed; then they can move us into a place where we can find what's important and right for us. Then we can assimilate them, take what is useful and supportive, and eliminate the rest. Once we are aware, understand, and listen to our guts' wisdom, we can make decisions and choices that are healing and supportive to our guts'—and our entire beings'—health.

There is a story of the disciple who went to the master and asked for his words of wisdom:

> "Could you tell me something that would guide me through my days?"
>
> It was the master's day of silence, so he wrote on a pad of paper, "Awareness."
>
> When the disciple saw it, he said, "This is too brief, can you expand on it a bit?"
>
> So, the master took the pad and wrote, "Awareness, awareness, awareness."
>
> The disciple said, "Yes, but what does it mean?"
>
> The master took the pad yet again and wrote, "Awareness, awareness, awareness means AWARENESS."

Awareness is the key. No one can show you what is hidden within, because only you know what your deepest self is all about. What you do not understand, you repress. When you understand, feel, and then let go, you can then make new choices and allow healing to occur. Here are some ways to invite awareness:

- Listening, embracing, communicating.
- Warmth on the abdomen.
- Deep breathing.
- Diet changes.
- Colonics.
- Cleanses.
- Belly massage.
- Movement.
- Journaling.

(See Chapter 8 for more detailed information).

When one is pretending, the entire body revolts.

—Anais Nin

Our mental, emotional, spiritual, and physical selves all interconnect. When we deny our guts' voice (our gut *wisdom*), we set up a conflict between our brain and gut that manifests itself as the gut's wisdom (symptoms). These "voices" are a blessing, offering you a warning to unhealthy eating and lifestyle habits. Unproductive thought patterns and toxic emotional holdings are often messengered to you via digestive and elimination distress, depression, and anxiety, as well as all other physical and emotional discomforts. As stated already in this book, stress-filled emotions have biochemical repercussions on our physical health, especially the reduction of our immune function. On top of that, I don't think I've met a depressed or anxiety-ridden person eating the healthiest diet. When we are upset, we seek out "comfort foods" that often contribute further to our guts' ailments.

Healing takes time to stop, listen, and make adjustments; healing is just another word for *change*. Personally, I love variety but disdain change. It's uncomfortable. It often takes slowing down. It requires effort and, oftentimes, courage. It's so much easier to pop a pill to rid ourselves of pain, learn to live with it, or hope when we wake up tomorrow it will be gone. However, when severe symptoms come knocking on your gut's door, the saying "if you have your health, you have everything" sounds truer than ever.

The body tells the clearest what we most want to hide.

—Marion Rosen

So the Gut Is the Messenger. What's the Message?

The message is this: Be aware; your wisdom is guiding you. The message is sometimes as simple as just listening and acknowledging your gut's need for dietary changes, a little stress reduction, down time, or some tender loving care. Its message may be assisting in discerning who or what is healthy for you. In other situations the messages may be connected to those deeply buried, "undigested," and unforgiven traumas or unhealthy attitudes and beliefs you carry within you. Without reflection on the whole "package"—gut, body, mind, and spirit—I believe one cheats him or herself of the full opportunity and experience of learning, growing and healing in the truest sense.

The "Payoff" for Not Listening

In his book, *Getting Well Again,* Carl Simonton, M.D., oncologist and author best known for his pioneering insights and research in the field of psychosocial oncology, states: "I believe we develop our disease for honorable reasons. It is our body's way of telling us that our needs—not just our body's needs, but our emotional needs too—are not being met, and that the needs that are fulfilled through our illnesses are important ones."

Angie, an attractive middle-aged singer, has been telling me for nine years that she'll get out there and audition once she feels better. She has experienced every kind of gut distress in the book, from uncomfortable gas pains to IBS. Always fearing something is more seriously wrong, she has gone from one doctor and healer to another, getting treatments and pills but few long-term benefits. As the years have passed, her symptoms have become more severe. She has shared with me that each practitioner has given her such love and care (which she doesn't receive from family and friends) and they are, in her words, "her dearest friends."

I am not dismissing Angie's abdominal distress. Her symptoms are very real, but they also have a very real benefit: Through these symptoms, Angie can receive the love and attention she's so desperate for. She can also avoid facing her fear of sharing her beautiful voice with the public.

In *Getting Well Again,* Stephanie and Carl Simonton, M.D., share their observations on why their patients became ill. They:

- ▷ Received permission to get out of dealing with a troublesome problem or situation.

- ▷ Got attention, care, and nurturing from people around them.

- ▷ Got an opportunity to regroup their psychological energy to deal with a problem or to gain a new perspective.

- ▷ Gained an incentive for personal growth or modifying undesirable habits.

- ▷ Didn't have to meet their own or others' high expectations.

Messenger Awareness

Spend a moment reflecting. What is your messenger speaking to you?

This should be done without any judgment. This is an opportunity to deepen your awareness of self and decide if there is an opportunity to make better choices—or not.

It's important that we don't deny, ignore, or medicate our guts in an attempt to get rid of uncomfortable symptoms that carry our guts' messages. Our guts need to be listened to, cared for, and respected, and one of the easiest ways to start respecting your gut is to pay attention to what you feed it.

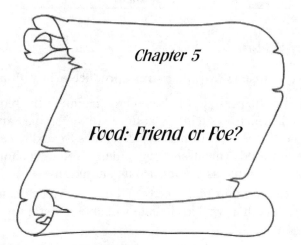

Chapter 5

Food: Friend or Foe?

What is food to one man may be fierce poison to others.

—Roman poet Lucretius

> The food choices you make can make or break me. I beg of you to choose wisely. As your biochemistry alters with each thought, emotion, or action, so it does with the foods and substances you ingest. You do not realize the power of foods to heal me, alter me, or even hurt me.
>
> Be a friend and eat friendly foods!
>
> —Your Gut

Ahhh, food. For a few of us, food is simply fuel. For a few more of us, food is a pleasure we enjoy with friends and family. And for some, food is a source of emotional comfort, eaten when upset, angry, or sad.

A delicately orchestrated symphony of biochemical changes occurs within us with each bite of food. Through the process of digestion, from organ systems to organs to cells to the reaction and action of molecules, our bodies are altered.

Molecules make up the cells that are the required building blocks of our organs. Molecules provide the fuel that each cell needs to carry out their specific jobs.

By choosing a healthy diet, we provide our bodies with the proper molecules that will reward us with optimum health.

Acid and Alkaline

Worry, anxiety, fear, and stress produce acid within us.

For health to be present, the body must maintain the bloodstream at a 7.4 pH level, which is slightly alkaline. All vegetables and fruits are highly alkaline. If the blood's pH level becomes to acidic, health is jeopardized. Protein foods (meat and eggs), dairy, soda, alcohol, sugar, and coffee are acid-forming, as are most nuts and grains.

In order to maintain balance, your body will leach calcium out of your bones and teeth as well as deplete valuable mineral reserves to neutralize excess acid.

To achieve a proper balance, the choices we make are important. I've labeled foods "friendly" or "foe" depending on how supportive they are to the balance of your body and gut's health.

A "friendly" food is a food that leads the gut to peace—freedom from indigestion, constipation, and other gut distresses. Friendly foods leave you energized and nourished. An "unfriendly" food is a food that can contribute to or cause gut ailments, such as bloat, gas, constipation, heartburn, irritable bowel syndrome flare-ups, and a myriad of other bodily and emotional discomforts.

If the foods that you eat are unfriendly, you may experience:

> Digestive disturbances including bloat after meals, gas, constipation, diarrhea, irritable bowel syndrome, nausea, indigestion/heartburn.

> Mental or physical fatigue, particularly after eating meals.

> Water retention (edema), where you lose or gain a couple of pounds in a single day.

> Food cravings and/or addictive eating.

> Frequent headaches.

> Skin irruptions (acne, rashes, psoriasis, eczema).

> Chronic pains in the form of muscle aches, pains, or arthritis-like symptoms.

> Emotional, mental, and behavioral symptoms, such as mood swings, irritability for no apparent reason, inability to concentrate, anxiety, and depression.

Many "unfriendly" foods are foods to which we may be allergic or have a sensitivity, and this can contribute to an array of physical and emotional symptoms.

Food Allergies and Sensitivities

For 12 years, Mary had severe migraines that landed her in the emergency room almost monthly. She was willing to let go of her wine, her chocolate, and her dairy, she was willing to go through a series of colonics and do yoga three times a week, but she would *not* let go of wheat, which was a food to which we suspected she might be allergic or sensitive. After working together for more than a year, she left discouraged. Mary called four months later to tell me that she had finally given in and surrendered her wheat foods. Her migraines stopped and have not returned!

Food Allergies

Food allergies are adverse immunological responses and systemic reactions to foods that other people can eat without any reaction. When you are allergic to certain foods or substances, your body has an antibody reaction to those foods in the same way it would react to germs or "invaders." Your immune system generally goes to war to destroy the invaders. Classic allergic symptoms that most are familiar with are sneezing, hives, rash, runny nose, headache, and gastrointestinal upset. These reactions can be triggered by dust, pollen, animals, and certain foods. Immediate, dramatic reactions such as a person's throat tightening after eating peanuts are the ones that most people associate with classic food allergies, but these account for only 5 percent of adverse reactions to food. Allergies can be easily detected by your healthcare provider through the use of patch skin tests and/or RAST blood testing.

Food Sensitivities

What happens when you eat a food you are sensitive to?

Frequently undiagnosed by conventional allergists, food sensitivities are a major reason why millions of us go through life with chronic gut ailments and other physical complaints. Food sensitivities may be at the core of a multitude of digestive and elimination challenges, as well as other physical and emotional symptoms.

Food sensitivities are usually triggered by common, everyday staples such as milk, corn, wheat, yeast, sugar, and caffeine. Because these foods are often eaten daily, a person may not be aware of their adverse effects on the system. Food sensitivities may show up as symptoms anywhere from two to 72 hours after ingesting the foe substance. This makes a sensitivity a lot more difficult to detect than a classic allergy. For example, you may eat whole wheat toast on Monday but get the bloated belly and achy muscles on Wednesday. Reactions such as bloat, irritable bowel syndrome, heartburn, and a host of other digestive and elimination ailments are common, but what many don't realize is that a food sensitivity may be the root cause of other symptoms, such as arthritic pain, weight gain, migraines, emotional mood swings (from depression to hyperactivity), and persistent food cravings.

A food sensitivity occurs when an enzyme deficiency causes us to be unable to digest particular foods. Large amounts of undigested proteins, fats, and so forth are left undigested, and the immune system treats these molecules as potentially harmful or toxic substances. As these larger molecules pass through your gut's lining, your supportive and protective immune system sees these molecules as "foes" and attacks them. An immune reaction is set into motion and an inflammatory response occurs. This response can contribute to inflammation and irritation within the gut (colitis, Crohn's, IBS) and show up as symptoms such as headaches, muscular pain, fatigue, and edema. Your body's wisdom attempts to reduce the irritation by retaining water, which dilutes the concentration of the offending toxic material. Tissues of the intestinal lining swell with protective water. In addition to a swollen intestinal lining, add gas formation from the putrefaction and fermentation of poorly digested food, and you have a gut that can make you look and feel months pregnant. Many people also experience daily fluctuations in weight. This is not a pleasant experience but a good way to detect a food sensitivity.

None of us are too happy with pants we can't zip up, but you must remember that the wisdom of the gut is actually protecting us from excessive toxins and possibly even more debilitating symptoms. Our guts are showing us quite vividly and uncomfortably that something we are ingesting is not okay within us.

And there's more:

> ⊳ Food sensitivities can cause serotonin levels to drop. Serotonin is a calming neurotransmitter that, when imbalanced, can lead to depression and anxiety, which can then lead to continued eating or "stuffing" ourselves with more inappropriate food. Serotonin imbalances have been implicated in cases of irritable bowel syndrome and other gut ailments.

> ▹ Your blood sugar levels drop, which can make you fatigued, shaky, moody, and hungry for something to boost you up. At this time, one might gravitate towards sugary foods or caffeine, which just continues the cycle.

> ▹ Food cravings and addictive eating occur. Certain food sensitivities can cause a release of your very own opiates. You can literally become addicted to the "high" your food sensitivities cause and seek out the offending food in order to get a "fix." Research from the *New England Journal of Medicine* (volume 337, 1997) states that opiate chemicals may also increase our appetite.

Food sensitivities can be detected by blood testing for IgG or IgG4 antibody reaction, or you can listen to your gut: Remove the offending food for 7–10 days. Your symptoms should calm down. Continue the journey of healing your digestive and elimination system with the befriending information provided within this book. In time, your body may balance toward a healthier state; therefore you may be less reactive to many of your previous food sensitivities.

The upcoming chapters will support you in correcting your gut's imbalances. Choosing the proper foods for your gut is one of the more empowering steps in your healing journey. Following are 21 befriending food gestures designed to help you discern the "foe" from the "friendly" foods. This will guide you in making wise food choices.

Befriending Gesture #1: Explore Other Grains

Despite the recent flood of low-carbohydrate diets, Americans love bagels, breads, donuts, and cakes. Breads are the "staff of life," so they say.

But the "staff of life" can hit you right in the gut and contribute to many a bloated and ailing belly. "But I eat *whole wheat* bread," I hear, and see a baffled and confused face looking back at me. High on the food sensitivity list is *wheat*. Wheat is found everywhere and under many other names: semolina (most pastas), durum, couscous, wheat germ, bran, graham flour, and farina. Wheat is also hidden in many processed foods, gravies, candy bars, processed luncheon meats, and creamed soups.

If you are sensitive or allergic to wheat, there is a possibility you may be also reactive to oats, rye, barley, and, in lesser amounts, spelt, due to the fact they all contain a reactive substance called gluten. Gluten is a protein, a sticky glue-like stuff that binds and holds grains together. (Gluten adheres to the bowel in the same sticky manner.) Gluten sensitivities can show up as mild symptoms of abdominal bloat, stomach upset, and runny nose to symptoms mimicking irritable bowel syndrome, headaches, migraines, joint and muscle pain, asthma, eczema, and mood swings. Serious digestive health challenges such as a condition called Celiac Sprue may be present. With Celiac, the villi of the small intestine are destroyed, which can lead to severe malabsorption of nutrients. This leaves one with a compromised immune system, weight loss, diarrhea, and fatigue.

Whether you have a sensitivity to wheat, other grains, or gluten, it can show up at the core of many digestive and elimination challenges, as well as a wide range of other health problems. I often say, as long as people are stuffing themselves with bagels, breads, and refined flour products (pastas, pastries, and cakes), I will have a robust business.

Whereas wheat or other food allergies can be detected through an allergy test, gluten sensitivity is difficult to detect with the typical tests. Although your doctor may be able to conduct allergy antibody tests or an intestinal biopsy, the easiest and least invasive way to see if you are sensitive to wheat and/or gluten is to *omit* gluten grains/flour products and replace them with brown rice, corn, millet, soy, quinoa, and amaranth. Then, let your gut speak to you. Wheat and gluten sensitivity seems to be fast-growing as we are exposed to chemically altered, refined, depleted, and processed foods. Even a small amount can cause a reaction. Your local health food store carries cereals, pastas, breads, bagels, and crackers, all of which are gluten-free. So there is no need to feel deprived. Read labels to make sure that wheat or gluten hasn't been slipped in.

Wisdom Tip

✦ In order to become aware of the cause and effects of gluten and suspected "sensitive" grains, *totally* omit them for seven to 10 days. Reintroduce them into your diet and then listen to your gut. (See Appendix C for a list of companies that make gluten-free products.)

Befriending Gesture #2: Eat 4 Servings of Veggies Per Day

At the top of the Gut Wisdom Friendly Food List, veggies are rich in antioxidant nutrients (cancer fighters). Cruciferous vegetables contain a substance called indol. Indols stimulate the production of certain enzymes that may help detoxify potential carcinogen. They are high in vitamins and minerals that build and restore your system. Because of the alkaline minerals in vegetables, they help restore the body's alkaline level to a healthy level. Their chlorophyll (the green in green vegetables) content neutralizes toxins that your body can do without. They are nonputrefactive, easy to digest (for most guts), and easily combined with most other foods.

Green leafy vegetables are an excellent source of absorbable calcium. (For example, two-thirds of a cup of collard greens will give 91 percent of the calcium in one cup of milk.) Vegetables are also high in fiber, which helps sweep food through your digestive tract. These guardian angels of fiber and nutrients have your best interest in mind, protecting against cancer, ulcers, and constipation.

Wisdom Tips

❧ On the top of the vegetable list to choose from are the cruciferous vegetables: broccoli, brussels sprouts, mustard greens, cauliflower, cabbage, spinach, and kale. Also include other "friendly" vegetables: carrots, lettuce, cucumbers, celery, squash, peppers (green, yellow, and red), string beans, yams and sweet potatoes, eggplant, and avocado. Try a variety throughout the week.

❧ Raw vegetables are an essential source of enzymes that aid digestion. However, individuals with weak or sensitive digestive tracts often find it difficult to digest raw foods. Slightly steamed, grilled, or baked vegetables may be best for those with a sensitive system. Try both and listen to your gut to see which satisfies it and agrees with it.

❧ Organic vegetables have been found to be considerably richer in nutrients as well as free from toxic pesticides and herbicides. Vegetables and fruits should be 80 percent of the diet.

Befriending Gesture #3: Eat 2 Servings of Fruit per Day

Fresh fruits are cleansing to the digestive tract, and are easy to digest and metabolize. Fruits are rich in bioflavonoids (flavonids). Bioflavonoids support the healing properties of vitamin C to fight infection, strengthen the walls of the capillaries (often recommended for hemorrhoids and varicose veins), provide antioxidant cell protection, and also act as an anti-inflammatory agent within the body. They are a rich source of complex carbohydrates, natural sugar, minerals, vitamins, and fiber. Their alkalizing effects may help reduce cravings for sweets.

Many fruits are rich in soluble fiber called pectin. Pectin helps you absorb calcium. Citrus fruits, figs, kiwi, and apples are an especially good source of pectin. Pears, peaches, plums, nectarines, and grapes are also good sources of vitamins and fiber. Melons, berries, cherries, mangos, and papaya are nutrient-rich. Bananas, tropical fruits, and dried fruits should be consumed in moderation by those sensitive to sugar.

Wisdom Tips

- Variety is the spice of life, so explore new fresh fruits and enjoy!

- Canned fruits are cooked, devoid of nutrients, and often processed with sugar. This turns a friendly food into a foe food.

- Choose organically grown fruit for your gut and body's health.

Befriending Gesture #4: Juice It up as Often as Possible!

Fresh raw fruit and vegetable juices are healing nectars. They are chock-full of mineral enzymes and antioxidants. There is no pill that can substitute for this friendly nectar.

Juicing your fruits and vegetables is a great way to add them to your diet. Plus, no processing or cooking has altered their cleansing and healing attributes. Ideally, drink an 8-ounce glass of raw vegetable juice and 8 ounces of fresh fruit juices a day. *Your gut would appreciate the company of these juices as often as possible.* Why not just buy bottled juice? Bottled juices, even those labeled "natural," are often made from concentrates, diluted with water, and packed with extra sugars. These juices have little nutritional value when compared with fresh raw juices. The benefits of fresh raw juices include:

- Cleansing and rebuilding of your gut.

- Instant energy. Raw juices need virtually no digestion, so the juices are easily absorbed and utilized for your healing.

- Moving toxins and waste from your body.

- Providing a plethora of nutrients that promote a strong immune system.

Each vegetable and fruit juice has its own unique nutritional effects on the body. Following are some of my favorites:

Cereal Grass

Wheat grass juice is abundant in alkaline minerals. Therefore, it is beneficial for overly acid body conditions such as candida overgrowth, chronic fatigue, and allergies. Wheat grass is not a source of gluten, so it is safe for wheat-sensitive individuals. Wheat grass assists in cleansing the blood, organs, and gastrointestinal tract. It is extremely rich in chlorophyll, which protects you from carcinogens and detoxifies the liver (the liver filters out stored internal toxins caused by stress and external toxins). Wheat grass stimulates the metabolism, and it is also a natural appetite suppressant. It can be taken in tablet form but is most effective when consumed fresh in juice form. The suggested amount is 1 to 2 ounces.

Vegetable Juices

▶ Carrot: Very high in vitamin A as well as rich in other vital vitamins and minerals; helps soothe and tone intestinal walls; cleanses the liver to discharge stale bile and excess fats; stimulates digestion.

▶ Spinach/Kale/Parsley: Rich in vitamins and minerals; all are high in chlorophyll, which increases bowel peristalsis and cleanses the liver, kidneys, and urinary tract.

▶ Ginger: Neutralizes toxins; aids in digestion, absorption, and elimination; stimulates elimination of mucous; increases bile secretion, which supports elimination and antioxidant protection for the liver.

▶ Beetroot and tops: A very powerful intestinal cleanser as well as blood-building juice; has been used to treat constipation, gall stones, anemia, and cancer (use mixed with other juices).

▶ Cabbage: Probably the least tasty of the juices, but contains healing properties for stomach and intestinal ulcers.

Wisdom Tip

↳ A favorite juice for newbies is carrot, spinach, apple, and ginger. As you acquire a taste for this gut-soothing nectar, add greens such as kale, beet leaves, and parsley.

Fruit Juice

Just about any fruit can be made into a delicious, as well as therapeutic, healing nectar.

▶ Apple: Eliminates toxins and is instrumental in enhancing the production of friendly bacteria.

▸ Grape and Grapefruit: Known to help cleanse the liver, which in turn has healing benefits for your intestines.

▸ Lemon: The fruit highest in vitamin C (move over orange!); increases bowel function and is believed to prevent gall stones (use one part lemon to three parts water).

Wisdom Tips

🍃 Fruit juices help cleanse your body and nourish it with rich, cancer-fighting antioxidants, but they are naturally high in sugar, so you "sugarholics" focus on green vegetable juices. And if your gut is a gas creator, cut out the fruit juice (and those smoothies, too!), as too much natural sugar could add to gut fermentation, contributing to your gut's distress.

🍃 Many health food stores now have juice bars. Experiment with different varieties. You may be surprised by how tasty fresh vegetable and fruit juice is and how good you and your gut feel afterward.

🍃 After experimenting with a variety of fresh fruit (and vegetable) juices at your local juice bar, you may consider purchasing a juicer for home use. (See Appendix C for a juicer recommendation as well as juice recipe books.)

Befriending Gesture #5:
Snack on Nuts and Seeds Between Meals

Nuts and seeds are a rich source of amino acids (protein) and essential fats and minerals. You say, "Goody, goody, I can eat nuts." Yes, but ideally eat nuts that are *soaked*; otherwise they can be difficult for most systems to digest. The second best way to eat nuts is raw or dry-roasted. Avoid nuts and seeds that are coated with sugar or salt. You can find nuts that have been seasoned with tamari (made from soy), which adds a pleasant salty taste.

Wisdom Tips

🍃 To soak your nuts: Cover the nuts with water and let them soak overnight in the refrigerator. Drain. Keep refrigerated and eat. If this doesn't grab you and you must eat roasted nuts, then chew, chew, chew, and chew some more to help assist in the digestive process. Listen to your gut.

- Nut Choices: Almonds, pecans, walnuts, cashews (high fat), Brazil, filberts(hazelnuts), chestnuts, macadamia, pine nuts.

- Seed choices: Sunflower, pumpkin, and sesame (contain an abundance of calcium).

- Nuts are great snacks in between your meals or garnishes on salads and vegetables.

- Avoid peanuts and peanut butters. Some peanuts have mold called aflatoxin that can potentially be toxic to your system.

- Explore nut and seed butters made from cashews, almonds, or sesame seeds (tahini). They are delicious substitutes for peanut butter.

- Though the fats in nuts are nutritious, eat nuts and seeds (and butters) in moderation unless you are trying to put on a few pounds.

Befriending Gesture #6:
Enjoy Eggs in Moderation (2 Eggs 3 Times Weekly)

Their reputation has been tarnished over the past few years due to the fact that they were associated with high levels of cholesterol. But we know that high blood cholesterol is only one indication of a high risk of heart disease, and that could be due to heredity more than diet. Researchers have found that we get only 25 percent of our cholesterol from what we ingest, and that the remaining 75 percent is produced by our own livers.

The fact is that, although egg yolks are rich in fat, they are also high in lecithin, which breaks down fat particles. Thus these substances balance each other out. They are also an excellent source of protein that can be easily utilized by your body.

I must caution against using commercially raised chicken eggs versus free-range organic eggs. Commercially raised chickens are pumped with hormones to stimulate growth and production of eggs as well as antibiotics to prevent disease. They are also crammed together in cages and never see the light of day. These are not happy chickens. Think of the stress-induced toxins being released. This all ends up on your breakfast table—a foe food, unless you choose free-range organic eggs.

Wisdom Tips

- ⚘ As with any food, enjoy eggs in moderation (two to three times a week).

- ⚘ Choose poached, boiled, or hard-boiled eggs

- ⚘ Try substituting tofu in place of eggs. Tofu has a similar consistency and will take on the flavor of your favorite seasoning.

Befriending Gesture #7: Reduce Consumption of Red Meats and Replace With Poultry, Fish, and Soy Products

A slab of prime rib makes many grin from ear to ear, but I'd like to share a few words of caution before you take a bite. Red meat is difficult to digest, causing it to linger longer, putrefying (rotting) in our gut. As you now know, this causes toxic bacterial imbalances and gut challenges. Most Americans ingest way too many meat products, which are acid-forming within our body and contribute to many of our health challenges. At breakfast, there's sausage and bacon; at lunch, hamburger and deli meats; at dinner, steak and ribs.

On a high-acid diet—more meat than vegetables and fruits—your system can become mineral-deficient. Minerals are needed to neutralize the excess acids in the blood, instead of doing their normal functions. The major acid-neutralizing minerals are calcium, potassium, magnesium, and sodium.

Calcium deficiency can result in osteoporosis, muscle soreness, and irritability. Calcium also plays an important role in cancer prevention. Calcium combines with harmful bile acids and fatty acids so they can get passed out of your gut before causing irritating effects on your gut.

A deficiency of potassium can contribute to bloating, infections, and heart irregularities. Magnesium deficiencies can result in elimination ailments, nerve problems, and weak bones and teeth. A shortage of sodium can result in digestive disturbance and weakness.

Meats contain saturated fats. Saturated fat contains a substance called *arachidonic acid* that encourages inflammation within the body. High intake of meat places undue stress on your liver. Meats also contain hormones, antibiotics, pesticides, and preservatives that are often added in breeding and processing.

Meat does contain protein and B12 but no fiber, which can contribute to constipation. Therefore, the more meat present in your diet, the less calcium there is available for absorption, which means your gut is less protected. Is this the job of a friend or a foe?!

Wisdom Tips

ᴪ Experiment with substituting the following for red meat: chicken, fish, turkey, eggs, soy products (tofu), beans, brown rice, legumes, nut butters, and unsweetened yogurt. Choose chemical, antibiotic-free foods. Most health food stores will carry an array of safe foods to select from.

ᴪ Have meat as your side dish and vegetables the main course, which helps you achieve a proper acid/alkaline balance. This will also help you not feel so deprived.

ᴪ Listen to your gut: Meat may agree with your system, leaving you feeling grounded and energized after eating. If this is so, enjoy it in moderation. However, if it feels like a rock in your stomach and you *still* want to eat it, then use a comprehensive digestive enzyme tablet (see "Befriending Gesture #20: Use a Digestive Enzyme With Your Meals," page 95) with your meal to assist digestion.

Befriending Gesture #8: Eat Fish, but Be Selective!

Fishy fishy in the brook, daddy catch him by the hook,
mommy fry him in the pan, baby eat it like a man.

That's a little song Dad sang to us some 30 years ago when basically all fish were considered friendly foods. On the friendly side, fish is a good source of easily digestible protein, low in cholesterol, as well as low in saturated fats. Cold-water fish (ocean fish) is a rich source of omega-3, an essential fatty acid found and needed in our brain cells, nerve synapses, and adrenal and sex glands. Plus, omega-3 can help lower cholesterol. Cold-water fish also have a high concentration of selenium (a mineral) that binds to toxins the fish ingest and basically renders them harmless.

Shellfish and fish from questionable lakes and rivers are foe fish. These types of fish can be imbued with toxins from their polluted water homes. "Mollusks that filter water such as scallops, mussels, clams and oysters can concentrate pesticides up to 70,000 times the concentration of sea water," says Elizabeth Lipski, M.S., C.C.N., author of *Digestive Wellness*.

Wisdom Tips

ᴪ Include fish in your diet two to three times weekly.

ᴪ Focus your intake on cold-water fish such as sardines, mackerel, salmon, halibut, tuna, and herring.

- If you don't know where the fish came from, don't eat it.

- Avoid raw fish (sushi). Parasites are easier to get than you realize.

Befriending Gesture #9: Beans Are a Great Fiber Source

When you join beans with a whole grain, you get a plant source of essential amino acids—or, in laymen's terms, a complete protein. Conscientious vegetarians use this combination as the heart of their meatless meals. Beans are both nutrient- and fiber-rich, however, they are generally difficult for many to digest, so they are often gas-producers.

Some tasty choices in the legume family are split peas, chick peas, navy beans, kidney beans, lentils, black beans, black-eyed peas, and soybeans (tofu, tempeh).

Wisdom Tips

- To make beans more digestible and less gas-forming, soak your beans overnight, drain the old water, replace with new water, then cook for several hours.

- Begin by including legumes in small portions to allow your gut time to get used to this high-fiber food source.

- Use Beano, an enzyme product, or ginger tea, to help digest and reduce gas incurred by these delectable friendly foods.

- For delicious, nutritious, meatless meals using beans and grains, a list of cookbooks can be found in Appendix C.

- As you experiment with bean cuisine, listen to your gut. Does this extra fiber please it?

Befriending Gesture #10: Substitute Soy, Rice, and Cultured Products for Dairy Products

Contrary to the claims of our milk-mustached celebrities, dairy products are not the friendliest foods. Dairy products can interfere with the gut's healing processes because of its high saturated fat content. Humans were never meant to consume anything other than human breast milk. Our digestive enzymes are not capable of breaking down a food that is meant to nourish another species. Up to 70 percent of Americans have an intolerance of dairy that can cause or contribute to poor digestion, gas, bloat, diarrhea, allergic reactions, and abnormal sinus phlegm and mucous build-up, thus clogging our gut's elimination system. Mucous clogs the intestinal villi that are needed for absorption of precious immune building vitamins and minerals.

Studies have also shown that dairy contributes to irritable bowl syndrome, ulcerative colitis, and Crohn's disease. These studies prompted the *New England Journal of Medicine* (1984) to state that "a physician should always consider the possibility that milk and milk products may be responsible for a patient's digestive symptoms."

Milk has been marketed as *the* calcium source. Actually, the body's ability to absorb milk proteins is quite poor because of the processing and pasteurizing. Hormone residue, antibodies, and additives from cattle-raising practices also hinder calcium absorption. You may say, "But where will I get my calcium?" Well, let me share with you some very healthy, absorbable, non-mucous-forming alternatives so that you do not fear sunlight shining through your porous bones!

Some great sources of calcium are leafy green vegetables, mustard greens, bok choy, kale, collard greens, sesame seeds, almonds, sunflower seeds, tofu, and sardines.

Wisdom Tips

- Some tasty dairy alternatives are rice milk, soy milk, and almond milk.

- Lowfat cottage cheese and goat cheeses can be tolerated by most, but soy cheese is a better choice.

- Eat butter in moderation.

- Now, here's the exception to the rule: *Cultured* milk products contain live healthy microorganisms that "pre-digest" lactose, which is the sugar in milk that so many have difficulty digesting. Products such as buttermilk, acidophilus milk, kefir, and especially plain yogurt can be tolerated by most. (The Hunzas who lived to be 100 years old knew something!) Yogurt is a good intestinal protector that contains friendly bacteria and vitamin A, vitamin D, and some B-complex vitamins. However, stick to plain yogurt, as those fruit yogurts are often filled with sugar, which only counteracts the benefits, leaving you with gas (foe) instead of gut ease (friend).

Befriending Gesture #11:
Avoid Hydrogenated and Saturated Fats

Fried chicken, potato chips, pastries, bacon, luncheon meats, ice cream, French fries, and cheese are all a big part of the American diet. Maybe you feel that you are a bit more progressive and joined the "lowfat" chips and yogurt craze.

We've heard a lot about the need to reduce the fat in our diets due to the belief that dietary fat may contribute to clogged arteries and cancer. When we eat fat, both of our brains release endorphins (feel-good hormones) and may lead us to crave even more fatty foods, especially if our essential fatty acids are too low.

Despite fat's terrible reputation, we do need a certain amount of fat in our diets. Fat provides energy essential to our immune system, our metabolism, and our ability to heal and helps produce needed hormones. Fats are needed to build and repair cellular membranes, especially in brain, nerve and white blood cells that keep inflammation at bay. However, we do need to pay attention to the *type* of fats we eat.

Foe Fats

▸ **Hydrogenated Fats:** Hydrogenated fats are found in fried foods, margarine, cakes, cookies, crackers, breads, cereals, some baby formulas, and most processed foods. Hydrogenation is a process in which unsaturated fats are converted into solid vegetable shortening. This results in the formation of transfatty acids that cannot be digested by our bodies. Hydrogenated fats are used in foods because they are inexpensive to use, they do not become rancid, and they allow for an extended shelf life. This reminds me of a nutritionist who brought a 7-year-old Twinkie with her to her nutrition lecture as a "hydrogenated showpiece." The Twinkie was fine, but the cellophane wrapper had slightly disintegrated. Our poor gut—what we ask it to try to digest! Transfatty acids are "stickier" than unsaturated fats, increasing the likelihood of plaque deposits in the arteries and liver. They have also been implicated in causing blood platelets to adhere together, thus increasing the risk of strokes and heart attacks.

▸ **Saturated Fats:** Saturated fats are found in foods such as dairy products, beef, and pork (including bacon). Saturated fats, besides being cholesterol contributors, are health hazards. Research has shown that saturated fats are a potential contributor to colon cancer. Our liver secretes bile, which carries our toxins (from foods, medications, the environment) out into our intestinal tract to be eliminated. If we are ingesting too much fat, our bile acid secretions can increase in the colon. Couple that with a lack of fiber (which carries out bile) and our daily gut stressors, and we end up with excessive levels of bile, which can be gut-irritators and tumor-promoters.

Are You a Low-Fatter?

Many lowfat products are now laced with synthetic fats. These are primarily being used in snack foods. Eating synthetic fats reduces the levels of fat-soluble vitamins (A, D, E, and K) in the body, which we need for a healthy functioning system. Synthetic fat cannot be broken down by our gut's enzymes; therefore it can't be absorbed and often causes a case of loose stools. This is why packages of synthetic fat-laced products often have this warning: "Caution: May cause digestive problems or loose stools."

Real fat slows down digestion and make you feel full longer. In the *Vitamin Bible*, Earl Mindell writes that some studies have indicated that individuals who substituted 20 percent of their fat with *fake fat* substitutes were not only ravenous by the end of the day, but they wound up eating almost two times their normal amount of fat-filled foods the next day!

My wisdom suggestion is that anything that causes vitamin depletion in our bodies, diarrhea, or gut disturbance, encourages us to eat more junk food with the illusion that eating it won't make you fat, *and* has a warning attached to it is *poison*. A foe food if ever there was one!

If you're looking to reduce your intake of dietary fat, I encourage you to go the old-fashioned route: Lower your fat intake by just cutting back on highfat foods.

Friendly Fat

We do need *natural* fats from foods such as fish, fish oil, seeds, nuts, and seed oils (for example, flax seed oil). These all contain important nutrients called essential fatty acids (EFA). Our bodies do not create EFAs, so we need to be conscious and bring them into our diets. EFAs are friendly fats! EFAs are broken down into two categories: omega-3 and omega-6. Together, omega-3 and omega-6 help in the creation and balance of prostaglandins. Prostaglandins are produced by every cell in your body, and they:

> ▶ Control inflammatory reactions.

> ▶ Strengthen the immune system.

> ▶ Protect your stomach and intestinal mucosal lining.

- Help eliminate food cravings and longing.
- Support proper liver function.
- Improve digestive function.
- Reduce PMS symptoms.
- Protect the heart.

Severe EFA deficiency can manifest as or contribute to irritable bowel syndrome, headaches, depression, anxiety, dry and patchy skin, and food allergies.

Omega-3 is found in tuna, salmon, mackerel, sardines, rainbow trout, pompano, canola oil, and primrose oil. Flax seed oil is one of the best sources of omega-3 fatty acids. A substance found in flax oil called lignans has been reported to block the growth of cancerous tumors, reduce inflammation, and help normalize hormone levels. This plays a key role in the prevention of colon, breast, prostate, and uterine cancers.

Omega-6 is found in sesame oil, flax seed oil, wheat germ, sunflower oil, and olive oil. Olive oil can raise levels of good cholesterol, which in turn can lower your risk of your "ticker" (heart) failing.

Wisdom Tips

- When purchasing oils, you want an oil that is labeled "unrefined" and/or "cold pressed" or you'll end up with an oil that has been bleached, deodorized, and filled with chemical solvents—not your gut's best friends!
- For optimum health, supplement your diet with essential fatty acid, omega-3 and omega-6 capsules daily.

Befriending Gesture #12: Wean Yourself Off Caffeine

Salivary glands ooze even with the thought of creamy milk chocolate or the smell of freshly brewed java, but the common denominator—caffeine—does not serve our gut's health.

Caffeine is a substance found not only in coffee and chocolate but also in black tea, colas, aspirin, and diuretic pills. Here's the friendly news: Caffeine stimulates the production of serotonin, our natural feel-good chemical, which is a brain transmitter produced by tryptophan. Serotonin gets our gray matter perked up. If the early morning has you a bit sleepy or grouchy, a caffeine "fix" can improve your mood and increase alertness by releasing adrenaline into the bloodstream (not bad for you in little doses). Caffeine has been used—moderately—for centuries for its therapeutic benefits.

The "Foe" News

▸ Caffeine can produce oxalic acid that hinders calcium absorption.

▸ Excessive amounts of caffeine can exhaust the adrenal glands, the organs that secrete adrenaline (our fight-or-flight hormone). This hormone lets us push a little harder, lets us work a little longer, and denies us the opportunity to listen to our gut wisdom, which may be saying that it's time to rest and take a breather. Over time, pushing our fight-or-flight button can lead to other hormonal imbalances as well as adrenal exhaustion—which means we're tired all the time.

▸ Caffeine has been indicated as the culprit in PMS symptoms, hypoglycemic imbalances, bladder infections, and gut imbalances, such as irritable bowel syndrome.

▸ Caffeine is a thief of B vitamins; it leeches them from the body. We need our B vitamins for healthy digestion, for elimination, and to keep our nerves calm. For many, caffeine (especially in coffee) may irritate the mucosal lining of our intestines, as well as the lining of the stomach, contributing to ulcers.

▸ Caffeine is a diuretic, which means it will draw water out of your body and gut, leaving you with dehydrated, hard stools (constipation).

▸ Coffee is a very acidic beverage and it can lead to an imbalance of friendly vs. unfriendly bacteria, which, as you know by now, is a condition that causes a host of gut disturbances: irritable bowel syndrome, constipation, colitis, candida, and so forth. Decaffeinated coffee (with the exception of Swiss water processed) can be even more injurious due to the chemicals used in the decaffeinating process.

▸ Some research has observed that drinking two to three cups of coffee per day may elevate blood pressure and increase the body's production of a stress hormone known as cortisol.

Wisdom Tips

↳ Try carob instead of chocolate. At least try!

↳ Cafix or Postum are coffee substitutes made from grains and have a reminiscent taste of coffee.

↳ Try an herbal pick-me-up such as ginseng, which is an herbal tonic to strengthen the body, not stimulate it. Peppermint or licorice tea is a delicious replacement.

- For the coffee-aholic: Begin by cutting back one cup at a time. Cut your cup with half-decaf (Swiss water processed). Begin replacing usual cups with tasty herbal teas, *Cafix,* or Postum. Green tea is very healthy and still offers a small "buzz."

- Learn relaxation techniques, such as meditation, deep breathing, and yoga, to help you get through the withdrawal symptoms that may occur (headaches, the jitters, anxiety, irritability).

- Be aware of the voice of the gut. Are your gut symptoms improving as you make these different choices?

- Journal as you are "getting off" caffeine. What feelings arise that caffeine may have been suppressing? This is an opportunity to do some emotional exploration and healing.

Befriending Gesture #13: Shake the Sugar Habit!

Sucrose, white crystalline sugar, maltose, dextrose, corn syrup, fructose, honey, maple syrup. *Oh, how we love it!* How we crave it, and how we get addicted to it! It has been noted that, in the United States, each person consumes an average of 130 pounds of sugar a year, which breaks down to about 1/3 pound daily. Many sugars are hidden. For instance, five to nine teaspoons can be hidden in your sodas. Cold cereals—the ones for children and especially the low-fat ones—can contain as much as 65 percent sugar. Catsup, salad dressings, mayonnaise, lunch meats, alcohol, and low-fat foods all contain sugar.

Sugar is a foe substance. It may offer us some immediate comfort during emotional periods, but in the long run it is a thief in our bodies. The list is long but worth mentioning. Excess sugar:

▶ Suppresses our immune system: 1/2 cup of sugar leads to a significant drop in phagocytes, the white blood cells that eat up harmful bacteria and are required for a strong immune system—impairing its ability to fight infection and disease.

▶ Causes our pancreas to secrete abnormally large amounts of insulin, which can be a major factor in hypoglycemia and diabetes.

▶ Feeds our unfriendly gut bacteria, adding to gut putrefaction and fermentation, setting us up for bloat, gas, and constipation.

▶ Steals our vitamins and minerals. Sugars take from our bodies because they themselves have no nutritional value. Sugars need our nutrients to be metabolized in our bodies, leaving us depleted.

▶ Robs B vitamins, which are needed for proper digestion and calmed nerves. It upsets the body's mineral balance, particularly calcium.

▶ Produces an overly acidic condition within the body that results in the stiffening of joints and muscles and digestive problems.

▶ Feeds candida, which has a direct effect on digestion. (See Chapter 10 for more information.)

▶ Makes us feel "out of touch," "spaced out," unfocused, and confused. This keeps us from listening to our gut's wisdom.

▶ Creates a false energy lift; keeps us trapped in a vicious cycle. When we eat sugar, we get a quick boost of energy, and our blood sugar rises rapidly. Our body then rapidly releases insulin, forcing the blood sugar level to plummet. The end result? You get shaky, fatigued, maybe even depressed. Another sugar "fix" is needed to boost you back up!

▶ Is empty nutritionally but abundant in calories.

Wisdom Tips

🍃 Artificial sweeteners may be FDA-approved, but there are still controversies concerning their safety. Sorbitol is another popular sweetener than can contribute to bouts of diarrhea. Personally, I'd choose pure sugars and natural alternatives rather than artificial (honey, maple syrup, stevia).

🍃 Use stevia as a sweetening substitute. Known as "the sweet herb," stevia is 25 times sweeter than sugar, non-caloric, and indicated as safe for people with candida and sugar imbalances such as hypoglycemia and diabetes.

🍃 Nibble every couple of hours on anti-sugar foods such as raw vegetables, nuts, seeds, fruits, hard-boiled eggs , chicken, fish, and/or vegetable juices (high in green veggies) in order to keep your blood sugar levels in balance and your cravings in control.

🍃 Steer clear or reduce intake of carbohydrates such as breads and pastas, which are converted into sugars in your gut and then instigate further sugar cravings.

🍃 Keep a food diary of everything you ingest. Becoming aware and conscious of what and how much sugar you are (unconsciously) eating. This is a great wake-up call to see how much sugar you unknowingly ingest daily.

- Exercise. Everything from walking to all-out aerobics will help control blood sugar swings.

- Read about candida (in Chapter 10), which is a gut imbalance that thrives on sugar for its survival.

- Think about where you are not receiving "sweetness" or goodness in your life. Begin observing this lack of "nourishment." How can you replace or begin to open up to this necessary and desired "nutrient" in your life?

- Be aware of and listen to your gut's wisdom. Are your gut's symptoms shifting as you let go of sugar?

Befriending Gesture #14: Decrease Alcohol Consumption

A little mind-/mood–altering libation from time to time is certainly pleasurable, but the consequences of overdoing it or drinking consistently can be immense. Alcohol is a drug, a foe substance that has negative effects on a sensitive gut, as well as negative emotional and mental effects. Alcohol contributes to:

▶ Malnutrition by inducing loss of appetite and/or by encouraging poor food choices that lead to vitamin and mineral depletion.

▶ Vitamin B complex depletion. These digestive supportive vitamins are used to metabolize the alcohol.

▶ Malfunctions in our central nervous system, the heart, brain (both of them!), stomach, intestine, pancreas, and liver.

▶ Imbalances of precious gut flora. The friendly bacteria gets killed, leaving you with an unguarded gut, which can then lead to diarrhea, irritable bowel syndrome, gas, bloat, candida, and increasing food sensitivity.

▶ The release of excessive gastric acid, which can cause irritation to the stomach lining, contributing to ulcers and the exacerbation of many other digestive problems you may already have (such as indigestion and heartburn).

▶ Low blood-sugar attacks. When blood-sugar levels are down, you may crave more alcohol and carbohydrates (pastas, pastries, bread, and sugar). Emotionally and physically, you may feel "down," thus perpetuating an emotional cycle of eating foe, depleting foods.

▶ Increased risk of cancer. For more than five decades research has associated alcohol with cancer, particularly of our gastrointestinal and respiratory tracts.

Wisdom Tips

🌢 Follow the Gut Wisdom Diet outlined in Chapter 6. Add or increase vegetables, whole grains and proteins, eat several (six) small meals throughout the day, and omit sugar and refined foods to keep blood sugar balanced to keep you properly nourished. This will lessen the physiological craving.

🌢 Supplement your diet with a good multivitamin mineral (with extra B complex and extra acidophilus and bifidus to replenish what has been lost).

🌢 What about wine? I know all about the research that concludes that a glass or two protects one against heart disease. I'm sorry to say that my experience with gut ailments has led me to say a big *no* to wine. Once clients remove wine (and beer) from their diets, significant gut health changes appear. If you need a little mind altering, try vodka, which is distilled from potatoes. The distillation process has agreed with more individuals' guts, rather than the fermentation process of wine.

🌢 Experiment by taking alcohol (a possible foe) out of your diet for a week (longer is encouraged). Listen to your gut. How is your gut responding to this change? Are there feelings surfacing that alcohol may have masked? Gently pay attention.

Befriending Gesture #15: Can the Soft Drinks

It's a multi-billion-dollar industry. Buy stocks in it; think twice about drinking it. Diet or regular, soda contributes zero nutrition to your system. It may serve as a comfort, filling you up in the short term, but it soon leaves you depleted and unnourished. This foe beverage contains phosphoric acid, carbonation, caffeine, sugar, or sugar substitutes. Take a look at what the sugar and phosphoric acid do: Both will cause your body's pH to plummet, leaching calcium from teeth and bones in order to buffer the acid/alkaline imbalance.

Carbonation in soft drinks increases the permeability of the blood-brain barrier. This barrier exists to protect us from toxic chemicals. When the barrier becomes more permeable, the chemicals from your soft drink (What chemicals? Just check the label!) reach higher concentrations in your brain. Carbonation enhances the chemical reactions from sugar, low-calorie sweeteners, and caffeine. Your liver must then work overtime to detoxify your body.

When ingested with meals, soda can lead to putrefaction in the gut, and that means gas and bloating.

If you feel bloated all of the time, your body may be retaining water. It is your body's way of trying to dilute the toxic substances from the soda to protect you from the soda's harmful effects.

Wisdom Tips

✦ Cut back on soda, or better yet omit it from your diet and replace it with mineral or seltzer water mixed with juice. Throw a lemon slice in your water.

✦ *E-mergen C* is a fizzy Vitamin C drink from Alacer. It is tasty, bubbly, and nourishing.

✦ If you are continuing to drink soft drinks, be sure to include a daily calcium and magnesium supplement to replenish the calcium-depleting effects occurring within your system from the phosphoric acid.

✦ Sodas found in health food stores are tasty and often sweetened with fruit juices and are much healthier substitutes.

Befriending Gesture #16: Say *No* to Processed Foods

Luncheon meats, canned foods, pastries, fast foods, white flour products, and so on have become staples for many. They've replaced our consumption of vegetables, fruits, whole grain and protein foods. They lack fiber, vitamins, and minerals necessary for optimum health. Processed foods are often laced with preservatives, excess sugars, saturated fats, gluten, salts, and unknown additives. In addition to them being nutritionally unsupportive of your gut's health, many people have allergic reactions to the preservatives and flavor enhancers (MSG, for example)—foe foods without a doubt!

Wisdom Tips

✦ Use fresh poultry and meats versus luncheon meats. Cook enough for the week ahead.

✦ If you don't have time to cook, explore health food store deli counters. They usually offer an array of freshly made, chemical-free foods.

Befriending Gesture #17:
Increase Your Water Intake to 8 Glasses Daily

Our bodies are 75 percent water. Each cell within us requires water to efficiently perform its job. When we are at our optimum of water intake our gut and body thank us. Water is critical to maintaining or achieving optimum health because:

▶ Every vitamin, mineral, amino acid (protein), hormone, and chemical messenger requires water to be carried to its destination.

▶ It is needed for every function of the digestive and eliminative systems.

▶ It prevents constipation and hemorrhoids by keeping your bowels hydrated and stools soft enough to move more easily.

▶ It (paradoxically) helps alleviate water retention. (You know, those swollen hands, feet, legs, and abdomen). When you are water-deficient your body perceives this as a threat to its survival and will begin to hold on to every drop. Diuretics offer only temporary solutions. The fluids are forced out along with some other vital nutrients. The body once again sees this as a survival threat and in its infinite wisdom will retain *more* water in order to protect you.

▶ It keeps your liver healthy. Water assists in flushing toxins out of your liver, which is the body's "oil filter," so to speak. A lack of water taxes your liver and contributes to fatigue, allergies, and poor digestion and elimination. Your metabolism becomes sluggish, and fat is stored in your body due to the liver's inability to efficiently break down fats.

▶ It helps prevent urinary tract infections by helping your body flush out toxins and harmful bacteria.

■ ■ ■ ■ ■ ■ ■ ■ ■

Which Water to Drink?

There has been controversy over which water to drink. Is purified water better than distilled? Is osmosis-filtered water cleaner than carbon-filtered? They all have their pluses, because they are all purified forms of water. I'll make it simple: Drink all water except tap water. (I suppose I should add don't drink from bubbling brooks or stagnant rivers!) Tap water can contain 500-plus chemical toxic substances. It also contains chlorine to kill the germs, but an accumulation of chlorine also kills the friendly bacteria in your digestive tract. There is a great deal of incriminating evidence against the safety of your tap water. Please choose purified water, whether you buy it bottled or you purify it yourself.

■ ■ ■

Wisdom Tips

↟ Your gut and body need approximately three quarts of "re-placement" water every day. Your foods can provide up to one and a half quarts or more—that is, if you are eating fruits and vegetables that are high in water content.

↟ Ideally, drink eight glasses of purified water daily.

↟ If you exercise, or it's a sweltering summer day, or you are consuming salt and/or salty food, your intake should be adjusted.

↟ If you are on a gut-cleansing regime (see Chapter 9), increasing your water intake is mandatory! Your gut needs plenty of water to assist in the removal of your waste and toxins out of your system.

↟ Carry a bottle of water wherever you go.

↟ Purified water is ideal for you, but if you dislike drinking water, try carbonated water. Or mix half carbonated water with half juice. Slowly wean off the juice and (gas-producing) carbonated water and drink straight, purified water.

↟ Toss a lemon slice in it for flavor and gut- and liver-cleansing benefits.

↟ Water at room temperature is best for the digestive process. Water too hot or cold alters the digestion process.

↟ Coffee and alcohol are fluids, but they can dehydrate your system because of their diuretic action.

↟ Juices and herbal teas are great but are not a replacement for the purifying action of water.

↟ If you believe you are hungry, you may actually be thirsty. Many of us mistake thirst for hunger, so we eat—maybe over-eat—to quench the unrecognized thirst. If you think you are hungry, drink a glass of water first and wait 20 minutes. If you are still hungry, eat.

↟ Listen to your gut and body. Check in periodically. Is it thirsty? Be a cordial friend and bring it some water. You'll go far with this gesture.

Befriending Gesture #18: Eat More Fiber Every Day

Fiber acts as an intestinal broom: It helps "exercise" the muscles of the colon, and it increases the bulk of your stool which makes your restroom experience easier and fulfilling.

Dennis Burkett, M.D., one of the first to research the benefits of fiber, performed an extensive study of Western diets high in refined low-fiber foods versus the rural African natives' high-fiber diets. His results: The high-fiber diets of the natives resulted in a quicker waste transit time (the amount of time that waste stays in the body) that was one-third the time of ours. The longer the waste remains in the body, the greater the chances of gut ailments occurring. Burkett published a paper, "Related Diseases—Related Cause?" in the respected medical journal *The Lancet* in 1969. He wrote that diseases of the intestinal tract, which are fairly common in our "civilized world," are virtually unknown in rural Africa. These diseases include colon and rectal cancer, hemorrhoids, appendicitis, diverticular disease, and polyps.

The National Cancer Institute recommends an intake of 20–30 grams of fiber daily. According to studies conducted by the USDA and the National Institute of Health, we consume on the average only about 12 grams daily. Start loading up on those fruits and veggies! Here are some of fiber's benefits:

> Fiber helps maintain a good "friendly" bacteria to "unfriendly" bacteria ratio with the gut, keeping dybosis at bay. Fiber is used by friendly intestinal bacteria in a fermentation process creating substances called short-chain fatty acids. One of these short-chain fatty acids is called butyric acid, which has been shown to stop the growth of colon cancer cells. Without sufficient fiber and friendly bacteria, this fermentation is halted.

> Fiber binds toxic and potentially carcinogenic substances (such as bile acids) and assists them out of the body before harm occurs. (Some bacteria in the colon can metabolize unabsorbed nutrients and by-products, such as bile, and transform them into cancer-producing substances.)

> Fiber absorbs and holds water, which can assist in keeping the stool softer, fuller, and easier to pass, increasing transit time and reducing toxicity.

> Extra bonus! Fiber binds to cholesterol and has been reported to reduce total blood cholesterol levels.

✿ Increase your intake of vegetables and fruits, legumes, and whole grains cereals and breads. If you are not getting sufficient fiber in your daily diet, add extra fiber in the form of ground flax seed, oat or rice bran, psyllium, or Metamucil to your diet daily. Fiber requires water to do its magic, so drink up. This is a wonderful addition to your wisdom program. *Avoid* wheat bran, as it can be irritating to many guts.

Befriending Gesture #19:
Protect Your Gut With Friendly Bacteria

They are our knights in shining armor, our gut's friend and protectors. Lactobacillus acidophilus and bifidobacteria (bifidus), the friendly bacteria, should be heavily populating our guts. When they are in short supply, putrefaction and toxic buildup occur in our colon. We become susceptible to illness and gut ailments caused by unfriendly bacteria and their chemical reactions within us. Acidophilus and bifidus are vitally important to our overall health. They are important for the proper function of our metabolism and digestion and for enhancing the protective defense mechanism of our immune system. They produce many of the essential B vitamins. They inhibit the growth of disease-producing bacteria and are essential for normal digestion and elimination.

Common symptoms associated with inadequate friendly bacteria are:

▹ Constipation.

▹ Gas and bloating.

▹ Bladder infections.

▹ PMS.

▹ Candida infections.

▹ Prostate inflammation.

▹ Vaginal infections.

▹ Skin conditions.

▹ Chronic diarrhea.

▹ Bad breath and body odor.

▹ Dairy product allergies or sensitivities.

▹ High cholesterol level.

An imbalance between friendly and unfriendly bacteria can be caused by many things, among them:

> ▷ Antibiotics and other medications.

> ▷ Oral contraceptives.

> ▷ Chemotherapy or radiation.

> ▷ Sugar.

> ▷ Foe foods.

> ▷ Stress.

> ▷ Poor digestion.

> ▷ Constipation (slow transit time).

The benefits of friendly bacteria are critical to the health of your entire body. Acidophilus and Bifido bacteria:

▶ **Restore and regulate your gut.**
Although they help to regulate proper peristalsis (bowel muscle movement), they are extremely useful for those who experience constipation and irritable bowel syndrome. They also prevent and treat antibiotic-induced diarrhea.

▶ **Aid in the production of lactase.**
Lactase is an enzyme necessary to digest milk and milk products (which are foe foods for many guts). Many people can begin to tolerate dairy moderately when they supplement their diets with friendly bacteria.

▶ **Are toxin eliminators.**
These bacteria deactivate various toxic compounds—such as nitrates—produced by other microorganisms or foods.

▶ **Are protectors of the immune system.**
These bacteria help stimulate formation of antibodies that prevent colonization of harmful microorganisms.

▶ **Improve nutrient absorption.**

> ▷ Heighten the protection against pathogens, viruses, and bacteria (flu, colds, food poisoning).

> ▷ Restore the gut's balance after antibiotics, medications, chemotherapy/radiation, poor food choices, and stress have altered the protective bacterial balance.

> ▷ Acidify the intestinal tract, which provides a hostile environment for microorganism and yeast (candida) to live.

> ⮞ Prevent overgrowth of harmful microorganisms such as candida, H-pylori, E-coli, and salmonella from taking hold in the gut and causing chaos.

> ⮞ Prevent urinary and vaginal infections from occurring or reoccurring (especially after taking antibiotics).

▶ **Are gas and bloat diffusers.**

Sufficient friendly bacteria helps prevent gases caused by putrefaction and fermentation. They are a gut toxin neutralizer.

▶ **Are breath sweeteners.**

When unfriendly bacteria are populating your colon, the gases produced by them can be reabsorbed into your bloodstream and carried to the lungs to be exhaled. Change the balance of your intestinal bacteria and your breath sweetens.

▶ **Aid with beautiful skin.**

As in the case of the lungs, toxins can also be carried to the skin, contributing to acne, liver spots, skin discoloration, and psoriasis. As the friendly bacteria reins, skin conditions often clean up.

▶ **Lower cholesterol.**

Studies have shown that friendly bacteria and a high-fiber diet can assist in normalizing cholesterol levels.

▶ **Aid vitamin production.**

Helps manufacture many of the B vitamins, which aid in digestion, and vitamin K, for natural blood clotting formation.

Wisdom Tips

⮞ Include daily supplemental acidophilus and bifidus capsules or powder for their prophylactic properties to ensure a protected gut (ideally a nondairy, refrigerated source).

⮞ Avoid the overuse of antibiotics or at least supplement with acidophilus and bifidus.

⮞ Eat daily or often a serving of plain yogurt (which contains friendly bacteria).

⮞ Follow a good diet (see Chapter 6).

⮞ Do the Gut Wisdom Cleanse. The ideal breeding ground for friendly bacteria is a clean colon. A constipated gut is an unfriendly bacteria breeding ground.

■ ■ ■ ■ ■ ■ ■ ■ ■

Do You Need Acidophilus and Bifidus?

❏ Do you have a history of antibiotic use?

❏ Do you have a history of corticosteroid use?

❏ Do you have a history of birth control pill use?

❏ Do you have bowel gas or heartburn after eating?

❏ Do you suffer from foul-smelling gas and stool?

❏ Do you experience constipation? Diarrhea? Irritable bowel syndrome?

❏ Do you suffer from allergies?

❏ Do you consume sugar, alcohol, coffee, or soda?

❏ Do you drink chlorinated water?

❏ Do you experience stress?

❏ Have you traveled to foreign countries?

❏ Do you use medications?

❏ Do you catch colds frequently?

❏ Are you lactose intolerant?

❏ Are you undergoing chemotherapy or radiation?

❏ Do you suffer from bladder/urinary tract infections or yeast/fungal infections?

If you said yes to any of these scenarios, begin taking acidophilus and bifidus daily to ensure a well-functioning gut!

■ ■ ■

Befriending Gesture #20:
Use a Digestive Enzyme With Your Meals

It is said that you are what you eat. I say you are what you absorb.

—Bernard Jensen, D.C.

We may get wiser as we age, but research shows that, as we grow older, our ability to produce digestive enzymes decreases. Enzymes are needed to break down (digest) the foods we eat into absorbable form. It is not only what we eat, but also what we absorb that keeps us healthy. Our gut manufactures a supply of enzymes as well as obtains enzymes from the food we eat (from foods in the raw state). As we age, poor food choices and stress often alter our ability to digest foods efficiently. This contributes to malabsorption of nutrients and, subsequently, can be a major contributor to many diseases. Good foods and nutritional supplements are of little use when there aren't sufficient enzymes to help break them down and assimilate them. Incompletely digested food molecules cannot be absorbed properly, leading to gut distress and allergic reactions. "One of the most important functions of enzymes is the conversion of our vitamins, minerals, and amino acids into vital neurotransmitters, allowing our bodies to function properly," says Louise Tenney in *Guide to Colon Health*.

If we eat in moderation, combine foods properly, eat nutritious foods, and process our emotional experiences, the body supplies us with the proper secretion of enzymes to digest our foods, and our gut runs smoothly.

The stomach secrets hydrochloric acid (HCl) for proper protein digestion; other enzymes are secreted into our small intestines for the digestion of carbohydrates and fats. When we are stressed, not eating correctly, and popping antacids and/or other medications, our enzyme activity can be altered. Enzyme production can also be inhibited by anger, worry, fear, and fatigue. The results can be:

> ▷ Indigestion (gas, bloat, heartburn), irritable bowel syndrome, constipation.

> ▷ Malabsorption of nutrients, which can manifest as lower immune functioning (more colds, flu, and so on).

> ▷ Heaviness in the stomach hours after eating (that is, food "sitting like a rock").

> ▷ Putrefaction and fermentation in the gut, which equates to bloat, gas and indigestion, and gut ailments.

> ▷ Fatigue after eating. Poor digestion stresses and overworks your entire system, leaving you feeling tired rather than energized.

> ▷ Undesirable bacteria and parasites can all enter and thrive in the digestive tract. Hydrochloric acid (HCl) in the stomach should have killed off these pathogens, but, if stomach digestion is inhibited due to stress, antacids, or medications, these critters can pass through and make a home in our guts, creating chaos.

> When food is not completely digested the gut responds to food residue as a foreigner or enemy. An inflammatory response can occur resulting in an irritated gut and food sensitivities.

Many of the approximately 90 million digestive problems Americans experience every year can be directly linked to poorly digested foods, says Lawrence Cheskin, M.D., director of gastroenterology at Johns Hopkins Bayview Medical Center in Baltimore. Everyone assumes that digestion just "happens." Well, not really. When our systems are compromised by stress, even the most pure, organic diet can't be put to effective use in our bodies.

Wisdom Tips

- Incorporate enzyme-rich foods into your diet: plain yogurt, kefir, miso, sauerkraut, and raw foods.

- Experiment with comprehensive digestive enzyme supplements with each meal. (You can find them in your local health food store.) They should include hydrochloric acid (HCl) to support protein digestion (unless you have been diagnosed with ulcers), lipase for fat digestion, and amylase for starch digestion. Vegetarian enzymes are also available to ensure an animal-free product. (See Appendix C.) Be consistent for a good period of time to notice the benefits and listen to your gut's praise.

- Chew, chew, chew. Chewing thoroughly allows enzymes contained in saliva to begin breaking down foods and stimulate the flow of gastric juices. Chewing activates a cascade of nerve and chemical responses that activates peristalsis (muscular bowel function). The yogis state, "Drink your solids, chew your liquids." Most of us take two or three chomps and gulp a drink to wash the food down. Attempt 10–15 chomps (a good yogi aspires to 30–50).

- Avoid drinking fluids with your meals as they will dilute your natural digestive enzymes. It is recommended that you drink fluids 30 minutes prior to and 30 minutes after your meal.

- Eat when you are relaxed, to ensure your meal gets digested well.

■ ■ ■ ■ ■ ■ ■ ■

Do You Need a Digestive Enzyme?

❑ Do you have gas and/or belching shortly after eating?

❑ Do you have gastric reflux/heartburn?

❑ Have you lost your taste for meat?

❑ Does food feel like a "rock" in your stomach even hours after eating?

❑ Do you experience constipation, irritable bowel syndrome, or other gut distress?

❑ Do you have abdominal bloat?

❑ Do you have a burning stomach that is relieved by eating?

❑ Do you have a whitish, coated tongue?

❑ Do you have a burning or itching anus? (This could also be parasite-related.)

❑ Do you have allergies or sensitivities to certain foods?

❑ Do you "inhale" your food?

If you are hearing these gut voices (experiencing these symptoms), it would be wise to experiment with a comprehensive digestive enzyme with each of your meals.

If you also experience lower bowel gas several hours after eating, be sure to also include acidophilus and bifidus as part of your gut care regimen.

■ ■ ■

Befriending Gesture #21:
Try Wisdom Food Combining; You'll Like It!

There are those lucky people who can eat anything, in any combination, and never experience the slightest heartburn, gas, or belly ailment. Most of us, though, experience uncomfortable symptoms such as constipation, irritable bowel syndrome, fatigue (especially after eating), and/or indigestion. Personal experience with clients has revealed that using food combining (and digestive enzymes) is a simple way to bring comfort to the gut's wisdom.

Food combining is based on the concept that different foods (carbohydrates, proteins, and fats) are digested by different enzymes and take different amounts of time to digest. When foods are improperly combined and not fully digested, putrefaction can occur, leaving the gut bloated, gassy, and overworked, thus leaving you feeling tired instead of energized after eating. The system then has to work harder to process and eliminate the overload. Improperly combined foods can leave one with any of the aforementioned conditions. Foods in proper combination, however, promote efficient digestion and elimination.

Other bonuses of proper food combining include: prevention of fermentation in the gut (which means less gas); a decrease in fluid retention; a reduction in allergies, indigestion, gas, heartburn, headaches, inflammation, and tenderness of muscles; and often even weight loss. Your gut won't have to work as hard, so you may experience more energy and less fatigue after eating, as well as more stable moods.

Here are some effective general guidelines to food combining. (For a comprehensive education of food combining, see *Fit for Life* by J. Diamond.) As you begin to experiment with food combining, maintaining a food journal is helpful to chart the results your gut reports back to you.

Wisdom Food Combining

▶ **Fruit:** Eat fruit alone. Eat fruit at least 20 to 30 minutes before your meal or two hours after your meal and approximately four hours after eating protein. If you eat fruit with your meal, it can cause fermentation and putrefaction (rot) that will cause gas and indigestion.

▶ **Vegetables:** Vegetables combine well with everything except fruit.

▶ **Proteins:** Proteins (eggs, poultry, beef, pork, fish, tofu) combine well with vegetables, so they can be eaten at the same meals.

▶ **Starches:** Combine starches (breads, pasta, beans, grains, potatoes, squashes) with vegetables in the same meal.

▶ **Proteins and Starches:** Proteins and starches or protein and fruits *should not* be eaten at the same meal, as they can't be digested efficiently together. The combination of protein and starch in the same meal causes food items to ferment and putrefy in the stomach, which leads to gas, bloat, indigestion, and other gut distresses.

▶ **Dairy:** Combine dairy with vegetables. However, if you are attempting to heal a digestive and elimination challenge, try to limit or totally avoid dairy due to the lactose sensitivities so many individuals experience as well as the mucous-forming side effects of dairy.

▶ **Other:** Sugars, coffee, soda, alcohol, and junk foods do *not* combine well with anything.

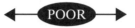

Food Combining
for Better Digestion

PROTEINS

Meats, fish, soybeans, most nuts, cooked or sprouted seeds (sunflower, sesame, pumpkin), eggs, milk (small amounts), cheese, yogurt.

STARCHES

Cooked or sprouted grains (brown rice, millet, buckwheat, oats, rye, barley), mature beans, potatoes, peanuts, chick peas, winter squash.

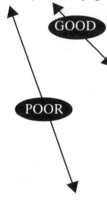

VEGETABLES

Leafy greens, seaweed, beets, carrots, asparagus, jerusalem artichoke, green beans, summer squash, turnips, radish, sweet corn, burdock, sprouts (mung, lentil, alfalfa, fenugreek), cucumbers (only with other vegetables)

FRUIT

Apples, pears, oranges, grapefruits, pineapples, lemons, bananas, dates, figs, dried fruit.

Wisdom Tips

- Remember not to drink any fluids 30 minutes before or after eating so as not to dilute your digestive enzymes.

- Chew, chew, chew.

- Eat in peace, without agitation or aggravation.

- Listen to your gut. If you feel full, stop eating!

- Remember to breathe. This slows down the pace of your eating and aids in digestion.

- Do your best with your wisdom food combining. Keep a journal. Try to properly combine foods at least one meal per day for a week. Listen to your gut. Continue proper food combining as you feel guided to do so.

In a Nutshell...

Here are the friendly foods that you can begin incorporating into your diet. If you suspect that you may have food allergies or sensitivities, it is gut-wise to omit these foes.

Vegetables (Low-Starch)

Leafy greens are high in calcium. These include spinach, collards, kale, bok choy, lettuce (avoid iceberg lettuce, which is devoid of nutrients), broccoli, celery, string beans, summer squash, carrots, celery, onions, parsley, cucumbers, asparagus, string beans, Brussels sprouts, tomatoes, peppers, sprouts. Vary your choices. *Avoid* canned vegetables with salt or additives and creamed vegetables.

Vegetables (High Starch)

Examples of high starch vegetables include sweet potatoes, potatoes, yams, and winter squash. Vary your choices; variety is the spice of life! *Avoid* canned vegetables.

Fruits

Apples, pears, kiwi, peaches, bananas, plums, grapes, pineapples, oranges, grapefruit, tangerines, berries, melons, and tropical fruits (mangos and papayas are examples). Fresh fruits in season are ideal. *Avoid* canned fruits, which are often artificially sweetened or laced with sugary syrups. Frozen fruits and vegetables are a fair alternative but will be lacking in many nutrients you can only obtain from fresh produce.

Dried Fruits

Eat minimally dates, apricots, prunes, cherries, raisins, currants, pineapples, and apples. Dried fruits are high in sugar and may be preserved with sulfites.

Grains

Examples include brown rice, corn, millet, amaranth, teff, quinoa, tritical, spelt, kamut, buckwheat, breads, crackers, muffins, pastas, cereals, and even cookies made from these grains (which can be found in your health food store). *Avoid* white flour products: breads, crackers, white rice, scones, cookies, cakes, muffins, and pastries; these are fiberless gut troublemakers. If you are sensitive to gluten, *avoid* wheat, barley, rye, and, to a lesser degree, oats.

Legumes

Black beans, navy beans, white beans, kidney beans, lentils, split peas, adzuki beans, chick peas, and soy beans (tofu) are examples of legumes. *Avoid* beans cooked with animal fat (such as refried beans) and canned beans with preservatives.

Fish

Broiled or baked fresh-water fish—salmon, halibut, trout, mackerel, herring, sardines, and tuna—are good choices. *Avoid* shellfish and fried fish.

Eggs

Ideally, eat soft-boiled, hard-boiled, or poached eggs fresh from free-range chickens. If you decide on an omelet, fill it with a variety of veggies. *Avoid* fried eggs.

Meats

Meats include chicken, turkey, lamb, and beef (in moderation). Available at your health food store are turkey bacon, sausages, and hot dogs. Meats are best if they are organic, free-range, and chemical-free. *Avoid* luncheon meats, hot dogs, smoked or pickled meats, fried meats, corned beef, and pork.

Dairy

Yogurt is the most digestible form of dairy. Feta cheese (goat or sheep's cheese) is also a good choice. Be aware that, for some individuals, dairy products can be highly mucus-forming, so it is best to *avoid* them during your healing journey. Try dairy substitutes such as soy milk and cheese, rice milk, rice ice creams, and almond milk. *Avoid* milk, cream, ice cream, and cheeses.

Nuts and Seeds

Raw or soaked nuts and seeds are best. Season with tamari. Good nut choices include walnut, pine nuts, pecans, almonds, macadamia nuts, cashews, Brazil nuts, and chestnuts. Enjoy nut butters from almonds, sesame seeds (tahini), or cashews. Good seed choices are sunflower, pumpkin, and sesame (garnish vegetables and salads). *Avoid* peanuts, peanut butter (very low quality), and salted nuts.

Beverages

Herbal teas (caffeine-free), fresh vegetable and fruit juices, and water are the best beverage choices. Water should be purified or distilled *avoid tap water*. Coffee substitutes such as Postum and Cafix can help coffee-lovers wean themselves off caffeine. *Avoid* alcohol, coffee, caffeinated teas, sodas, and sweetened juices.

Oils

Cold-pressed oils such as olive, safflower, sesame, soybean, sunflower, corn, and flax seed are quality choices. *Avoid* all saturated and hydrogenated oils.

Sweeteners

Natural sweeteners include real maple syrup, barley malt, rice, syrups, honey, stevia (a natural herb sweetener), and fruit-sweetened jams and jellies. *Avoid* sugar, corn syrup, sugar substitutes, and jellies and jams with added sugar.

Condiments

Examples include herbs and spices, tamari or shoyu sauce, Bronners Liquid Amino Acids, sun-dried tomatoes, anchovy paste, mustard, horseradish, Worcestershire sauce. Use butter moderately. For your salads, use health food store salad dressing or homemade dressings made from balsamic or rice vinegar, lemon, olive oil, and herbal seasonings. Avoid excessive salt.

■ ■ ■ ■ ■ ■ ■ ■

Befriending Gestures

- Vary food choices on a daily basis.
- Focus on alkaline-forming foods.
- Experiment with vegetables as your main course.
- Eat in moderation.
- **Avoid** liquids *with* meals.
- Explore wisdom food combining.
- Include acidophilus, bifidus, and digestive enzymes as needed.
- See the Gut Wisdom Diet (Chapter 6).

■ ■ ■

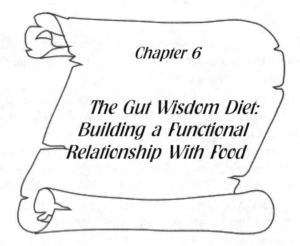

Chapter 6

The Gut Wisdom Diet: Building a Functional Relationship With Food

Habits at first are silken threads, then they become cables.

—Spanish Proverb

I am aching to be heard. I am burning to be listened to. My needs are simple. As you befriend me, I promise you won't even notice me.

—Your Gut

Months after a heartbreaking divorce, Carrie's normally reliable digestive system went completely haywire. Constipation, bloat, and dull, throbbing headaches became her constant companions. In an attempt to soothe herself, Carrie fed her gut "comfort foods": pizza, pasta, meats, mashed potatoes, wine. The more she ate, the worse she felt, and the worse she felt, the more she ate. After weaning herself from some of these "foe" foods and undergoing a series of colonics, she began to feel better. Encouraged by these results, Carrie learned how to breathe deeply into her gut, massage her abdomen, and apply warmth to her abdomen to comfort herself physically and emotionally. She practiced some forgiveness exercises and began to let go of the anger and hurt she'd been holding onto before and during her divorce. Carrie's system began to regain proper function, and her heart is on the mend.

One of the most important aspects, along with our food choices, is how we relate to food. Our relationship with food (in other words, our food choices) can offer us insight and awareness of ourselves. Once we are aware of how we choose to nourish ourselves and with what foods, what we attempt to bury and stuff within us, how we handle our stressors, and how tuned-in we are with our ever-present inner wisdom, we can start to be open to change.

Food and emotion have become intermingled within us since childhood. When we were fed by Mom and other loved ones, it was often as a source of love and nourishment. We got the ice cream cone if we were good, the hot cocoa if we were cold. After falling off our bicycle, we may have been consoled with a hug, a kiss, and a lollipop. Some of us were denied food as a means of punishment for some undesirable behavior; others were pacified with sweets as a substitute for love and attention. And let's not forget the always-popular guilt: persuading us to eat everything on our plates because of all the starving children around the world.

Over the years this ingrained training has caused us to use our foods not as a source of physical nourishment, but as a dysfunctional substitute for love, comfort, attention, and pain relief. As we become aware of the foods we choose, when we eat them, and the amounts we ingest, we can begin to explore what needs and wants are calling for expression and release and what foods are attempts to ease inner pain and emotional emptiness.

Our goal is respect and self-love, which is true nourishment. This sometimes-challenging feat can begin by befriending the gut's wisdom, thereby inviting a functional relationship.

With awareness, we can begin the journey of developing a functional relationship with our gut, our food, and ourselves. As with any successful relationship, listening is the key.

■　■　■　■　■　■　■　■　■

How to Develop a Functional Relationship With Food:
Listen to Your Gut!

1. Ask your gut what it needs to nourish it. With the knowledge you now possess, you will be able to use many of the befriending gestures to tap into your gut's wisdom.

2. Be *aware* of the reasons why you eat. Eating on automatic pilot does not allow you to hear and notice what the gut is saying back to you. Before you eat, get in touch with yourself. Eliminate outside disconnectors, such as television and radio. Close your eyes, place your hand on your abdomen, and take three deep breaths. Ask yourself: On a scale of one to 10, how hungry am I? How does hunger feel inside me? Am I eating because I'm lonesome, sad, angry? What am I not expressing or asking for?

What is not fulfilling in my life? What am I truly hungry for? Notice and become aware, and then choose your food. Are you energized or fatigued after eating certain foods? Are your digestion and elimination systems operating "happily," or are there voices of discomfort (indigestion, bloat, constipation, diarrhea)?

3. Be *aware* of foods that medicate you. Often we overindulge and use food to repress uncomfortable emotions. As you experiment with omitting foe foods, your gut's natural wisdom will allow these emotions to surface. Be observant and gentle with yourself as these arise. Allow yourself to feel them, grieve them, and let them go.

4. Are there foods that you are not willing to let go of? Don't judge yourself harshly. Simply notice it. Then, when you feel you are ready, omit one foe food at a time. Always replace it with a friendly food, so as not to feel deprived. If it is truly a struggle to let go of a particular food or substance, just let it stay in your diet for now. You will experiment or let go when you're mentally and emotionally ready.

5. The first few days and weeks of any changes are generally the most difficult because your body is *withdrawing* from many of its favorite "drugs" (sugar, caffeine, fast foods, fried foods, alcohol, and so on). Treat your body as a friend. Talk to it, explaining that you, too, have been uncomfortable, in pain, and so forth for too long and that it is time to find out what it is like to feel good.

6. Give yourself a "Treat Day." If you love chocolate, bless it. Eat it. Enjoy it.

7. Keep a wisdom food journal as you are experimenting with new food choices. Listen to your gut; it will speak to you and let you know whether a new food is friend or foe. With a friendly food, your gut will be free from symptoms. A foe food will have the gut speaking back to you with heartburn, gas, constipation, and other gut voices. Journal what emotions are present with these new changes.

8. After eliminating foe foods for a period of time you may choose to participate in the Gut Wisdom Cleanse (Chapter 9). The Cleanse will support you in discerning the cause and effect of the foods you choose.

■　■　■

The Gut Wisdom Diet

The Gut Wisdom Diet is an eating plan that integrates all the friendly foods and wisdom food-combining suggestions listed in the previous chapters. As you follow it you will find that you will not only experience better gut health, but more energy and a general sense of well-being. Don't be surprised if you lose a few pounds in the process! Listen to your gut, as you journey and experiment with the Gut Wisdom Diet.

Breakfast

One of the following:

> ▷ Fresh fruits (organic, if possible).

> ▷ Fruit smoothie.

> ▷ Baked apple sweetened with raisins and real maple syrup.

> ▷ Whole-grain (gluten-free) cereal (rice, spelt, quinoa, millet, or oatmeal) with rice, soy, or almond milk; add 2 tablespoons of ground flax seeds.

> ▷ Granola with rice, soy, or almond milk; add 2 tablespoons of ground flax seeds.

> ▷ Bread, muffins, or bagels (gluten-free).

> ▷ A protein drink.

> ▷ Soft-boiled or poached eggs or an omelet with vegetables.

> ▷ Gluten-free pancakes, waffles, or French toast with real maple syrup.

(See Appendix C for gluten-free products and cookbooks.)

Lunch and Dinner

▶ Salads with a mixture of five or more vegetables (excluding head lettuce, which has minimal nutrient value) and a dressing of olive oil, lemon juice, and/or herbs. Most health food stores offer a wonderful selection of salad dressings. Try different ones; variety is the spice of life! Add a protein to the salad: salmon, turkey, chicken, tofu. Enjoy a slice of gluten-free bread.

▶ Steamed, stir-fried, baked, or raw vegetables sprinkled with toasted sesame seeds. Squeeze fresh lemon over them, and drizzle with olive oil.

▶ Baked or broiled chicken, fish, turkey, or tofu with veggies and a salad.

▸ Brown rice/beans and vegetables.

▸ Rice, pasta, and vegetables.

▸ Burritos (corn) filled with vegetables and soy cheese or rice.

▸ Sweet potato with vegetables and a salad.

▸ Rice/spelt/amaranth pasta with vegetables and a salad.

▸ Homemade soups (without cream).

Snacks

▸ Fruits.

▸ Vegetables.

▸ Plain rice cakes or crackers.

▸ Nut butters (almond, tahini, sesame, cashew).

▸ Trail mix (nuts and seeds).

▸ Dried fruits.

▸ Plain yogurt (add fresh fruit and sweeten with stevia).

▸ Guacamole and corn chips.

▸ Popcorn.

▸ Deviled or hard-boiled eggs.

Beverages

▸ Herbal teas.

▸ Fresh vegetable juices.

▸ Eight glasses of purified water per day.

Wisdom Suggestions

↳ Invite a sense of awareness to each meal or snack: listen, ask, listen.

↳ Use *Wisdom Food Combining* as much as possible. (Refer back to the wisdom food-combining chart on page 100.) Listen to how your gut responds to these healthy, well-combined meals.

↳ Have vegetables as your main course. Include plenty of the green, leafy variety.

↳ Do not drink fluids with your meals.

✦ Don't eat when you're upset, worried, or angry. If you do, please remember your digestive enzyme, to help you digest your food, and apply warmth (Belly Buddy) to the abdomen while eating (see "Warmth" in Chapter 8).

✦ Breathe, chew, and be mindful of this important "taking in" process.

Supplement With:

▸ Digestive enzymes at each meal.

▸ Ground flax seed. Ideal once in the morning and once in the evening. (You can mix 2 tablespoons in a protein drink or juice, or on your veggies, in salads, or in cereals.)

▸ Acidophilus and bifidus daily (two capsules three times per day).

▸ Essential fatty acids (omega-3 and omega-6) (one capsule three times per day).

▸ Super Green capsules or tablets (two capsules three times a day).

And that's it! Remember that *any* positive change you make will benefit your gut and your body, so do not punish yourself if your diet isn't "perfect" or if you forget a supplement. You are trying to learn how best to nourish *your* gut and your body, and this can take time and patience.

Now that you understand what kinds of foods the gut likes best and the kinds of foods it doesn't, it's time to move on to those substances that can trouble it.

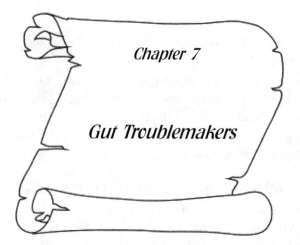

Chapter 7

Gut Troublemakers

The body, too, calls out for compassion; it doesn't want to be treated the way the polluters treat the rivers and the skies.

—Sy Sakransky

Here's something you've probably figured out as you've been getting acquainted with me: I'm sensitive. You would be wise to know what kinds of things cause me trouble.

When you use antibiotics, non-steroidal and steroidal medications, laxatives, and antacids, you change my healthy bacteria balance. Stress and negative thoughts and attitudes wreak havoc on me.

You probably just want the pain and discomfort to go away. You don't want to be inconvenienced, slowed down, or uncomfortable, so you may pop a pill. This can make it easier to ignore me but can injure me even more. If you want me to be quiet, find out what troubles me.

—Your Gut

The gut needs a proper amount of protein, carbohydrates, fats, vitamins, minerals, water, enzymes, and fiber to work efficiently. However, many of us add antacids, laxatives, or other medicating substances to our daily diets. (In school, I don't think we learned that Tums or Ex-Lax belonged to any of the basic food groups!) We want to eat what we want to eat, when we want to eat it, choosing not to believe that we are responsible for our gut voicing its opinion with acid indigestion, constipation, or other ailing belly voices. We may not realize that "self-medicating" is our way of ignoring health-directing gut messeges.

We also have not been taught the repercussions of "self-medicating." Nor have we been educated on exactly how damaging stress, our thoughts, and our emotions can be on our digestive and elimination tract.

Following is a list of commonly used medicating substances—as well as other gut troublemakers—and their effects on the gut.

Non-Steroidal Anti-Inflammatory Drugs (NSAIDs)

Pain is never pretty. It is a message from our bodies that something needs attending. While in the throes of pain, we may use anti-inflammatory medications to help bring us some immediate comfort. It is wise to know what gut troubles these medications will leave with you. NSAIDs are products such as aspirin, ibuprofen, Motrin, and Tylenol. These drugs are generally sold over the counter to relieve aches, pains, and inflammation. NSAIDs work in our body by blocking prostaglandin synthesis. Prostaglandins are small protein messengers found throughout our bodies. Some prostaglandins assist in healing and repair; others cause inflammation and pain. When you take NSAIDs, *all* prostaglandins are blocked; it's an all-or-nothing deal. Your immediate inflammation and pain are gone, but then your long-term ability to heal and repair is diminished. Taking NSAIDs:

> ⊳ May irritate and inflame the intestinal tract, contributing to food sensitivities, skin conditions, arthritis, and colitis.

> ⊳ Increases the risk of ulcers of the stomach and duodenum.

> ⊳ May increase gut permeability (leaky-gut syndrome). This allows toxic substances to cross the weakened bowel cell membrane into the bloodstream.

> ⊳ Continuous aspirin consumption can result in bleeding of the gastrointestinal tract (stomach, colon).

> ⊳ Can contribute to dybosis, an imbalance of friendly and unfriendly bacteria that can leave you vulnerable and unprotected from viruses and other disease-producing microorganisms.

Steroids

Cortisone and prednisone are emergency drugs used to treat chronic inflammatory conditions including arthritis, asthma, lupus, Crohn's disease, ulcerative colitis, psoriasis, eczema, and allergies. Steroids are very powerful anti-inflammatory drugs that reduce inflammation but that, over time, can cause severe side effects. The prolonged use of steroids:

> ▷ Can have many side effects, such as swelling of the face, hands, and ankles, as well as weakening of the joints, thinning of the bones, and ulcers.

> ▷ Can suppress the immune system, lowering your resistance to combat infections.

> ▷ Can feed and exacerbate candida (see "Candida Albicans" in Chapter 10), which further damages the intestinal lining and leads to other gastrointestinal and body-wide ailments.

> ▷ Inhibits your own natural anti-inflammatory chemicals (protoglandins), which can cause you to become dependent on the medication indefinitely.

> ▷ Can stress and damage the liver.

Antibiotics

My father may have been a bit dramatic when he called antibiotics "poison," but he may have known intuitively that the overuse of these medications was harmful in the long run.

Antibiotics have come to the rescue for many serious infections because they can kill off dangerous, harmful bacteria; I wouldn't want to have invasive surgery without an antibiotic available to protect myself. However, antibiotics are equal-opportunity killers. They kill off friendly, gut-protective bacteria as well as the harmful bacteria. Thus the overuse of antibiotics can encourage new infections, allergic reactions, diarrhea, constipation, stomach upset, and yeast overgrowth (candida).

It is now known that the indiscriminate and prophylactic use of antibiotics has caused some bacteria to mutate and become resistant to them. In 1995, the Center for Disease Control stated that only 50 percent of 110 million prescriptions for antibiotics may be appropriate for the illness being treated. A significant amount of antibiotics sold are given to animals raised for slaughter. So, as we chomp on our burger, steak, or chicken breast, we get a dose of antibiotics that can kill off the friendly flora in the gut and make us less resistant to harmful bacteria. The number of antibiotic-resistant bacteria is increasing worldwide and turning into a massive public health problem. There are now strains of bacteria that simply have no effective treatment to halt their invasion and may require aggressive treatments with powerful drugs that can be compromising to the immune system.

As these harmful microorganisms (bacterias) become more resistant to conventional treatments (antibiotics), the wisdom of our gut encourages a mandatory need for us to strengthen our immune system's function in order to keep bacteria infections at bay.

How to Replenish Friendly Bacteria During Your Antibiotic Treatment

This is such an important time to use the friendly bacteria (acidophilus and bifidus) to protect your gut (and your health) and prevent further complications. As you are taking antibiotics, follow this protocol:

Do not take acidophilus and bifidus at the same time you ingest your antibiotic. For beneficial results, take three capsules or 1/4 teaspoon powder of each approximately two hours after each antibiotic dose. After the antibiotic treatment is completed, take six capsules or 1/2 teaspoon powder daily for a period of two weeks to repopulate your gut with friendly bacteria. Thereafter continue with the recommended daily dose to maintain your newfound level of friendly bacteria.

Always used bottled or purified water. Tap water is highly chlorinated, which is helpful in killing dangerous bacteria but, unfortunately, kills friendly bacteria as well.

Laxatives

Are we a society that's "full of it"? Laxatives are a multi-million dollar business. According to the American Cancer Association, 20 million people use laxatives. Is this a comment on our society, food, and lifestyle choices? How are we handling our stress? How are we "holding on" and forcing out old toxic stuff (emotions and attitudes)?

Most chemical laxatives work by stimulating and irritating the bowel muscles to increase peristalsis (muscle bowel action). The bowel responds by attempting to remove the irritant, sometimes causing gripping and spasms.

Laxatives can be habit-forming. The chronic use of laxatives can abuse the bowel muscles so that they become lazy and dependent on their use—that is, needing more and more laxatives to continue to get the same effect. The excessive use can cause damage to the nerve cells in the colon wall, whereby one may need to retrain the bowels to have a bowel movement on its own. Laxatives can reduce the absorption of nutrients and deplete the precious mineral balance within our bodies. They will also alter the bacterial balance in the gut, which will lead to a compromised immune system and ripple into other health challenges.

Safe, bulking fiber products such as psyllium, Metamucil, and ground flax seeds increase the bulk of the bowel's contents and absorb water to make the stool softer. This gives the bowel muscles something to help them assist waste elimination *gently* without harsh irritants. However, you must take these products with plenty of water; otherwise you may experience further constipation.

There are also certain bowel toning and strengthening herbs, such as aloe vera, cascara sagrada, turkey rhubarb, dandelion, and buck thorn bark, which can be supportive for those who have misused or overused bowel-weakening laxatives.

The occasional use of a laxative is fine, but prolonged use can be habit-forming, damaging the overall health and strength of the gut. Most importantly, regularly using these products can mask deeper problems that need your attention, such as dietary or lifestyle imbalances, as well as emotional issues. What are you holding on to so dearly? (For further guidance, see "Getting off Laxatives" in Chapter 10.)

Antacids

My educated guess is that, if you are using antacids, your dinner tonight was *not* brown rice and vegetables. Call me a psychic, but you may be eating fast foods; overeating; drinking alcohol, coffee, or sodas; and eating when you are stressed.

Heartburn is caused by stomach acid backing up into your esophagus. About one-third of the U.S. population experiences frequent burning sensations, regurgitation, belching, and a sour taste in the mouth. This gastric reflux/heartburn has been on the rise over the past 20 years.

When diets are shifted to healthier, high-fiber choices and proper food combinations, the heartburn will often dissipate, a message perhaps that the trouble is not too much stomach acid but choosing the wrong foods in the wrong combinations repeatedly. Using antacids for a short period of time may be initially helpful, but prolonged use can create significant problems with digestion and microbial overgrowth.

Blocking your stomach acid with antacids without making other alterations has several negative side effects that the advertisers and even your doctors don't share with you: A gut with suppressed stomach acid becomes vulnerable to harmful microorganisms (bacteria, viruses, parasites). One of the jobs of stomach acid (hydrochloric acid) is to kill these unwanted predators—think of the guard at the door. So, microbes that you may pick up from eating at a restaurant where the cook, busboy, or waitress may have forgotten to wash her hands, or where the food was not cleaned thoroughly, may be passed on to you over your candlelight dinner. Sufficient stomach acid would have normally killed these microbes, but now the microbes have an opportunity to enter your gut, make themselves at home, and cause havoc.

Another job of stomach acid is to help break down certain nutrients for easy absorption, especially iron and calcium. Overusing antacids may set you up for calcium deficiencies such as osteoporosis and anemia. I know that advertisements say that *your antacid has calcium in it,* but calcium needs stomach acid to be absorbed properly! Stomach acids help digest protein. If your digestion is compromised, conditions such as gas, bloat, food allergies, and dybosis (a toxic gut) can develop from insufficiently digested proteins. Many antacids can be constipating, compounding the problem.

Many antacids contain aluminum, a toxic metal that has been implicated in conditions such as Alzheimer's, heart trouble, and pulmonary and bone disease.

Antacids often cause the production of even more acid, a condition called "acid rebound." In a natural reaction to the suppressed levels of stomach acid from the antacid, your stomach will secrete a double dose of acid to catch up with what has been suppressed. Hence you reach for another antacid. A vicious cycle is then created. This is a process similar to the suppression of emotions: When you suppress in order not to experience necessary feelings, those feelings eventually bubble up to the surface, distorted and exaggerated.

Do those vegetables and brown rice sound a little more inviting yet?

Not Listening to Mother Nature

When we don't honor the call of Mother Nature because we are too rushed, are too busy, can't or won't go to the bathroom in the department store, at work, or at our new date's home, we contribute to the dysfunction of the colon's job.

In *The Second Brain,* Dr. Michael Gershon tells a story to answer this question: Can the gut's brain learn and be trained? An old army sergeant, a nurse in charge of a group of paraplegics, would give his patients enemas at 10 a.m. every day so that they would not become constipated. The sergeant was eventually rotated off the ward, and his replacement decided to give enemas only after patients became impacted (severely constipated). But, at 10 in the morning, every patient on the ward had a bowel movement *without* an enema.

The gut is trainable. If we ignore the signals of Mother Nature, though, we confuse the gut and contribute to our discomfort. When waste reaches the lower colon (the sigmoid) and the rectum, it is about 70 percent water. (The remainder is bacteria, dead cells, food residue, and indigestible materials.) The longer it remains inside you, the more water will absorb back into your system, leaving dry, hard, and difficult-to-pass stool. Trying to pass a brick is uncomfortable as well as a contributing factor to constipation, hemorrhoids, and the proliferation of unfriendly gut bacteria.

"Transit time" is the time it takes between eating breakfast on Friday and when you finally flush on Saturday. Ideally the time frame should be from 24 to 36 hours. A delayed transit time could be a significant contributing factor to autointoxication, or self-poisoning. Inadequate fiber and water, poor food choices and combinations, food sensitivities, stress, and emotional "holding on" can contribute to slower transit times. On the average, Americans have a transit time that can range from 48 to 96 hours. This is a long time to not "take out the garbage!"

I've heard doctors say that it might be your body's "normal" rhythm to have a bowel movement every second or third day. I steadfastly disagree! Just because our diets and stress levels contribute to this sluggish transit time doesn't mean that it's normal! IBS, constipation, indigestion, colon cancer, and so on are *not normal.* They are the result of our neglect and lack of knowledge about the importance of moving our bowels.

■ ■ ■ ■ ■ ■ ■ ■ ■

Bowel Transit Time Test

Use activated charcoal tablets or caplets. Take five caplets. (Charcoal is occasionally used for temporary reduction of intestinal gas and can be purchased at your local drug or health food store). Jot down the time when you take charcoal. When the charcoal arrives in the toilet bowl, your stool will be colored black, and you will be able to calculate your own transit time!

Your grade: If the results show up in less than 12 hours, this is generally an indication that your foods are moving through you too rapidly. You may not be absorbing the nutrients from your foods, thereby not nourishing your body optimally.

If your results show up more than 36 hours later, this indicates that last year's Thanksgiving dinner may still be hanging out, increasing your risk of gut toxicity and an ailing belly.

If you "fail" your test, don't worry. Whatever the results were, there are ways to improve bowel function and create a healthier relationship with your gut. (See Chapter 10 to improve your transit time.)

■ ■ ■

Toxic Thoughts and Feelings

Stress: Our gut says NO, but our mouth says, 'I'd love to.'

—Dick Francis

You just *think* of your ex-spouse and your gut aches. You wake up anxious, wondering how you are going to pay all those accumulating bills. You are frustrated and fearful about your long, unsuccessful job search, and your gut tightens and constipates with the thought of another day in an unfulfilling, dead-end job. This, in a nutshell, is stress. When these emotional stressors begin to snowball, it can take a serious toll on the gut's health as well as the immune system.

"Once an emotion is created, it needs to be released or expressed or will become stress held in the belly or body," says Ken Dychtwald in *Bodymind.* If anger, fear, worry, and frustration are a constant part of our "emotional diets," they can become poisons that can eat away or fester within us, upsetting our guts' health.

As stated previously in this book, emotions are not just neutral notions; they alter our biology. As does a pharmacy, our cerebral and gut "brains" create and secrete an assortment of drugs (chemicals) that affect both our moods and biology. The mechanisms through which emotions such as anxiety, depression, anger, despair, joy, hope, and love can affect the gut's health are related to the autonomic nervous system and those tiny protein messengers called neuropeptides. When you are thinking positive thoughts, you're experiencing a sense of well-being, and your emotions (neuropeptides) are flowing and expressed, the body's chemistry is positively affected. When you are chronically stressed, angry, and unforgiving and when emotions are stuck and "held"—watch out!

It takes only a blink of an eye, whether you are *just thinking* about a stress-filled situation or actually experiencing it presently, for a chain reaction to occur within you.

The body's fight-or-flight response kicks in: The sympathetic nervous system pumps out stress hormones such as cortisol and adrenaline, heart rate and blood pressure increase, breath becomes shallow and rapid, and blood is diverted from the gut and pumped to other muscles to get the body ready to fight or flee. Meanwhile, the gut's natural function is put on hold until the "stress" subsides. When this occurs, digestion is altered as the body slows down important enzyme production. If the digestion process is not working properly to digest meals, the repercussion may be heartburn, gas, bloat, and other bowel irregularities. Intestinal muscles may slow down, causing constipation; may become stimulated, contributing to diarrhea, spasms, or cramps; or both—as in the case of irritable bowel syndrome.

The immune system is also affected. The stress hormones adrenaline and cortisol can contribute to other health conditions: headaches, ulcers, anxiety, stomach cramps, insomnia, fatigue, obesity, accelerated aging, and damaged brain cells. High cortisol levels have been indicated in cases of cancer.

■ ■ ■ ■ ■ ■ ■ ■ ■

You can eat a perfectly balanced diet, cleanse your body inside and out, and exercise religiously, but, if you are in a state of mental and emotional stress, your ailing belly and other health conditions in all probability will *not* go away.

■ ■ ■

Secretory IgA

Secretory IgA S(IgA) is an antibody that is a valuable component of the immune system and that is present throughout the entire digestive tract. It is our system's first line of defense against colds and flu as well as an overall indicator of the health of the immune system. Therefore, the higher the S(IgA) level, the stronger the immune system, which directly leads to a greater ability to resist disease.

"The Physiological and Psychological Effects of Compassion and Anger," by Glen Rein, Ph.D., Mike Atkinson, and Rollin McCraty, Ph.D., in the *Journal of Advancement in Medicine* (1995), shows the impact of one 5-minute episode of recalled anger on the immune antibody IgA over a 6-hour period. The slight increase in IgA that was initially recorded at the onset of the anger episode was followed by a dramatic drop—that persisted for 6 hours!

According to Mantak and Maneewan Chia's, *Chi Nei Tsong*: "The undigested traumas (i.e., grief, old hurts, resentments, sadness) in our lives collect in our gut as a knot. It will hold this trauma until it is safe to release it. The Taoist sages of ancient China observed 'energy blockages' in internal organs that result in knots and tangles in their abdomens. These obstructions occur at the center of the body's vital functions (our gut) and constrict the flow of chi affecting our body's immune function. The negative emotions of fear, anger, anxiety, depression, and worry cause the most damage. Always in search of an outlet, these negative emotions and toxic energies create a perpetual cycle of negativity and stress." Hopefully, you understand the impact stress has upon the body and the value of being aware of and managing our thoughts and expressing our feelings so they serve and honor the gut and body rather than harm us. Maybe think twice before getting angry with the crazy driver in front of you, worrying about finances, or holding a grudge against your ex!

■　■　■　■　■　■　■　■　■

Gut Wisdom

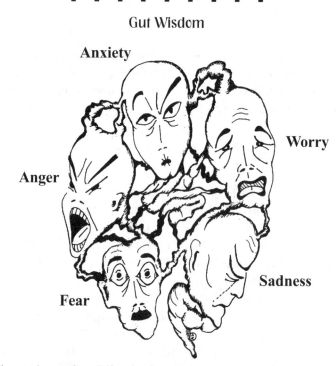

Our "undigested emotions" live in our gut:

> *If negative emotions can't find an outlet (cannot be expressed or let go of) they will fester in the organs or move into the abdomen, the body's 'garbage dump.'*
>
> —Chi Ni Tsang, *Internal Organs & Chi Massage*
> by Mantak and Maneewan Chia

■　■　■

Food Overindulgence

I never eat more than I can lift.

—Miss Piggy

Eating—what an ingenious way to distract and stuff feelings of anger, loneliness, frustration, and stress! Foods can numb us out and help us to avoid what we're feeling—temporarily.

Overeating puts our digestive and elimination systems into overdrive. Our systems weren't designed to work so hard. Excess mucous production (which leads to malabsorption of nutrients) may occur if our system gets overwhelmed by a barrage of chocolates, breads, steaks, dairy, pastries, and poorly combined multiple meals. Indigestion, constipation, bloat, irritable bowel, and weight gain are loud messages from your gut! They are letting you know that overindulgence may be taking its toll on you.

Sugar, pastries, alcohol, and sodas are all empty calories, stealing nutrients from our body in order to metabolize them. Many of the nutrients robbed from the body (especially the B vitamins) for processing "empty-calorie" foods are needed for well-functioning digestive and elimination systems and essential to our ability to handle stress. Sugar, breads (which turn into sugar in the system), and alcohol feed the *unfriendly* bacteria in our guts. This causes a fermentation and putrefaction process that can contribute to bacterial imbalance, leaving the gut unprotected from harmful microbes, and yeast overgrowth.

Alcohol, besides numbing you out, strips the gut lining of good bacteria, leaving it open for inflammation, irritations, and leaky-gut syndrome.

Coffee is the top of the list for the most frequently drunk beverage. Besides the caffeine exciting the nervous system—this is what causes many of us to visit the bathroom—too much coffee can cause intestinal spasms, bacterial imbalance, and irritation and can exacerbate an irritated bowel. Calcium and magnesium are lost with each cup. If ulcers are a concern of yours, coffee stimulates the flow of stomach acids, making matters worse.

With the excitation of the nervous system, we are generally not calm and centered in our bodies, leaving us disconnected from our feelings and important gut-wisdom messages.

Eat Only When You Like Him or Her

An important way of avoiding digestive trouble is to be *aware* of the mood you're in when eating. If you are eating when upset, angry, or frustrated, you are setting yourself up for indigestion, gas, and a slew of ailing belly complaints. For example, when you eat when you're angry, your nervous system flips into fight-or-flight mode. This bodily process shunts blood away from your gut to your muscles (so you have the strength to pick up your suitcase and run to your mother's!). Digestion slows down, as do other gut functions.

When you are relaxed—when you like him or her again—your nervous system shifts into the calm and restorative parasympathetic mode, your gut is receptive to food, efficient digestion...and a hug.

Chapter 8

Gut Befrienders: Creating a Functional Relationship

What you cannot find in your body, you will not find anywhere else.

—Asian Proverb

There are so many things that bring me peace and comfort. If you gift me with those gems, I can promise you that you will barely notice me except for the clear, subtle guidance I am constantly giving to you.

Along with the foods and substances you feed me and the stresses you release, how you breathe into me, exercise me, touch me, warm me, and listen to me all have a profound effect on how well I am functioning.

—Your Gut

A befriender is a trained listener for those in trouble, with physical and emotional pain—think of a Good Samaritan. Befriending is the intent of acting or being a friend. When one befriends, there is listening, caring, compassion, and a feeling of connection.

If we are not listening to our inner wisdom, we are not being a very compassionate friend to ourselves. We are disconnected. In our disconnection with self, physical, emotional, and spiritual blocks are created. Blockages prevent the life-giving flow of energy (life force), and blood to create whole-being health.

Within this chapter are many necessary gifts to give your gut to reconnect and assist it back to the road of health. Each one is worth experimenting with and implementing as new befriending habits.

Belly Breathing

Inhale...exhale...inhale...exhale. If you're like most people, you probably take the process of breathing for granted. Though it is an automatic function, improving upon it can help you befriend your gut and improve your health.

Our diaphragm does about 80 percent of the work of breathing. It provides the floor on which the lungs and heart sit and forms an arched dome over the liver, stomach, and intestines. When we are stressed, our breath is shallow (this is called upper-chest breathing). Our diaphragm tightens and is unable to do one of its other jobs: gently massaging the liver, stomach, and intestines; stimulating them; and promoting their natural functions. Our digestion and elimination functions are basically "out of commission" as our breath is restricted.

When we are relaxed and unstressed, our breath deepens into our belly. The parasympathetic branch of our autonomic nervous system begins to reign. Belly muscles relax, our diaphragm massages our internal organs, and digestion resumes. Belly breathing helps us slow down, helps us calm down, and allows our body to begin to restore balance within us. Belly breathing releases a variety of messenger molecules such as endorphins, our bodies' natural opiates, which help relieve pain and discomfort as well as alter our moods. Laboring women are often taught how to breathe themselves through the pain. Yogis use consciously controlled breath patterns to alter their consciousness into a state of blissful calm.

Why Do We Breathe Shallowly?

Emotions affect our solar plexus, a collection of nerves just below our diaphragm, which Eastern practitioners have often called "the seat of emotions." We automatically and habitually make our breath shallow—in other words, we tighten our diaphragm—so as not to feel the emotional stirrings within our gut. Unconsciously, we have learned to shut down these "gut feelings"; shallow breathing is a common physical response to anger, stress, fear, sadness, and pain. Do you remember crying freely as a child until an authority figure barked, "Stop that crying...or else"? In order to stop, you sucked up your breath, tightened your tummy, shut down the flood of tears, and stuffed the emotions within. We continue to do this when in stressful, uncomfortable, or frightening situations. We hold our feelings at bay while unknowingly disrupting our gut's function.

"The way we breathe has a profound effect on the way we feel," says psychologist Phil Noerenberger, Ph.D., author of *Freedom from Stress*. "Many stress-related complaints, whether physical, mental, or emotional, are caused by improper breathing. But fortunately, many of these complaints can be reversed simply by learning to breathe properly."

Take a Breather!

Under pressure? When stress builds, your neck and shoulders tense, and your head and gut begin to ache. Belly breathing can automatically take you out of the *stress response*. You can shift this damaging tension by breathing deeply and consciously, allowing your neck, shoulder, and abdominal muscles to relax.

Anxious? When your mind is chattering at a mile a minute, jumping from one thing to another, you're probably breathing rapidly and shallowly. Rapid, shallow breathing can cause fatigue, chronic anxiety, as well as feelings of disorientation. Allow yourself to relax and start breathing deeply into your belly.

Need anger management? When you're so furious that you feel as if you are about to explode, take very deep belly breaths. Make sure to exhale completely each time. Not only will you feel calmer, but you'll be better able to handle the issues that triggered your anger.

In pain? Cramps and bellyaches respond well to belly breathing. If deep breathing can decrease the pain of childbirth, then it can make a difference in any pain you may experience. Belly breathe right into the gut discomfort...and watch it disappear.

Toxic? You know that moving toxins out of your system is important. We eliminate up to 70 percent of toxins (carbon dioxide and other gases) through our exhalations. The more robust your breath, the cleaner your innards!

Wisdom Awareness Invitation

Notice when you are inhibiting your breath; is it:

> When you are driving in traffic?

> When you visit your in-laws?

> When you are looking for a new job?

> When you are at work?

> If your gut is in distress?

> While you are eating?

> ‣ When you feel fearful or anxious?
> ‣ When you are thinking about your ex?
> ‣ When you are standing in line in the grocery store?

I invite you to experiment with deep belly breaths when you experience tension, stress, and daily irritations. Belly breathing is a great stress-reducer, plus it is beneficial to your gut's health. A wonderful way to use breath is in the form of prayer and/or meditation. The word *spirit* comes from the Latin word *spiritus*, which literally means "breathe."

Here's how to start befriending your gut through belly breathing:

1. Lie on your back, wearing loose, comfortable clothing.
2. Place a Belly Buddy (see Appendix C for more information) or pillow on your stomach for visual feedback on the depth of your breathing.
3. Rest your hands on your belly, Belly Buddy, or pillow.
4. Relax and notice your breathing pattern as the pillow or Belly Buddy rises and lowers.
5. Inhale deeply through your nose. As you inhale, the downward movement of the diaphragm should press your abdomen outward. (With each inhalation, visualize air filling your lungs and abdomen).
6. Exhale out through your nose. Gently pull your abdominal muscles in as you exhale. Your abdomen should sink back down. *Try to find a breathing rhythm that feels comfortable for you. Notice your hands rising and falling as they rest on the pillow.*
7. Now, let's add a variation. Breathe in slowly to the count of eight. Hold your breath to the count of four, relaxing around the held breath. Exhale again slowly for the count of eight.
8. As you exhale, let go of all worries, concerns, and negative thoughts. Inhale peace and relaxation; all is well.
9. Repeat the breathing cycle five times. Feel the relaxation spread throughout your entire body.

Warmth

Warmth on your belly can feel like a comforting hug from a friend. It's like the soothing sunshine that melts tension away. It's like a hot bath that dissolves knots, aches, and stresses. This is one of my personal favorite ways to befriend the gut!

When you apply warmth to your ailing gut it helps draw blood to your abdominal organs to assist the healing process. (Remember that when we are stressed, blood is shunted away from our digestive and elimination organs, causing our gut to shut down.)

Warmth relaxes tight, spastic, and tense abdominal muscles. Warmth, because of its comforting nature, invites you to breathe deeply. This allows your restorative parasympathetic nervous system to respond by returning proper function back to your digestive and elimination system. Now, instead of ignoring, denying, or medicating your aching gut, you have the choice of bringing it soothing tender care. Use warmth to befriend your gut:

> ▸ After or during eating. This helps bring blood and circulation back to the gut encouraging good digestion.

> ▸ To soften tight abdominal muscles and ease bellyaches, cramps, spasms, constipation, IBS, and menstrual cramps.

> ▸ Whenever you feel digestive or eliminative discomforts.

> ▸ Before or after your belly massage (see "Belly Massage," page 128).

> ▸ During belly breathing exercises.

> ▸ To lull you to sleep.

> ▸ When your emotions and daily stresses have gotten to you.

> ▸ When you feel emotionally vulnerable and feel the need to protect or nurture yourself.

> ▸ Just because it feels good!

Befriending Invitation

You can place warmth on your belly using just your hands. Simply rub them vigorously together to create friction that will make your hands warm.

You may also use a warmed wash cloth, a Belly Buddy, a hot water bottle, or a heating pad. Preferably the heating pad is non-electric to prevent exposure to electromagnetic currents. (See Appendix C for information about the Belly Buddy, an easily-heated aromatic pillow for the belly).

Place one of these on your abdomen and breathe deeply into your belly. Listen to tranquil music. Notice how your belly likes this warm "hug." Good befriending points here!

Belly Massage

When you touch a body you touch the whole person, the intellect, the spirit and the emotions.

—Jane Harrington

The history of massage dates back to the beginning of time. Massage is touch. Since the beginning of mankind, the desire to touch and be touched, and indeed the *need* to be touched, has been embedded in the human psyche. Monkeys raised without mothers to hold and cuddle them grow up to be antisocial and aggressive. Babies raised in orphanages who were not physically touched and soothed often *died*, though they were clothed and fed.

When we were young and had a tummyache, Mom may have rubbed it lovingly to make it all better—and it worked. Now it's our turn to rub our bellies. Massaging the belly can release trapped gases and waste matter contributing to many of our belly ailments.

There are other added benefits—Mom intuitively knew. It turns out that touch stimulates our own healing feel-good chemicals from our *gut and brain*. The healing benefits of massage involve both the relaxation of the body and its positive effects on the mind. As tension is released, you feel better physically, emotionally, and mentally.

Our gut's brain and cerebral brain are ultimately connected and constantly affect each other. Our solar plexus is a collection of nerves just beneath the diaphragm near the stomach and liver. We often react emotionally in this area. This is often called the seat of the emotions. The belly can manifest issues about being nurtured and receiving physical, emotional, and spiritual nourishment. Tension in this area can contribute to constipation, ulcers, and female imbalances.

A bloated, hardened belly may serve as a type of armor and protection, shielding us from our vulnerable feelings or attacks from others. This armor of bloat, gas, and waste matter may also serve to deaden intense feelings manifesting after abortion, incest, rape, sexual harassment, painful childbirth, or abdominal surgeries.

As stated by Candace Pert in her book *Molecules of Emotions*, "When emotions are repressed, denied, not allowed to be whatever they may be, our network pathways get blocked, stopping the flow of the vital feel-good, unifying chemicals that run both our biology and our behaviors.... The body and mind are not separate, and we cannot treat one without the other."

Massage is a powerful gift of connection and healing. As you befriend and connect with your belly with massage, you may be assisting the release of trapped gasses or years of buried emotions. Massage with compassion and respect, for this area is both a vulnerable and a sacred area of unexcavated stories and feelings.

Befriending with a belly massage:

> Assists in dislodging trapped gases and waste matter.

> Is very beneficial in stimulating the blood and lymph circulation to rid the body of toxins.

> Relieves stress. (Therefore it strengthens resistance to disease and promotes wellness.)

> Relieves cramping.

> Helps move the *chi*. The better the flow of this energy, the better our emotional and physical health.

> Stimulates and regulates our natural chemicals, increasing a sense of well-being.

> Can be used to explore and release areas where you may be "holding" emotions, which may be manifesting as physical gut ailments.

> Feels good!

Befriending Invitation

As you massage each section of your belly, be aware of tight, tender areas. If emotions surface, allow yourself to feel them, continue to breathe deeply, then let them go.

1. Lie on your back with a pillow under your knees.

2. Pour warmed massage oil into the palms of your hands.

3. Take three deep belly breaths.

4. Starting at the lower right side of your belly, directly above the hip bone, move your fingertips in a circular motion, slowly moving up the right side until your fingers are just below your ribcage. Stop often to take a few belly breaths.

5. Continue to massage across your upper belly, just above your navel and down your left side to just directly above your left hip bone.

6. If you notice any tender or tight areas, apply light pressure with your fingers on that area and imagine your breath is entering into that space. Notice how that can relieve the discomfort.

7. Repeat the process once again, this time spiraling in toward the navel.

8. Complete the massage by placing both palms on the center of your abdomen and allow a deep belly breath to fill your abdomen.

9. Place a hot water bottle, heating pad, or heated Belly Buddy on your abdomen and notice how relieved your gut feels.

Brush Off the Past: Dry Skin Brushing

We lather our skin with lotions and oils to keep it moist and smooth. We use antiperspirants to prevent our skin from normally perspiring. As a result, our skin pores become blocked, and toxins and metabolic waste products become trapped in our bodies instead of being naturally released through the sweat glands. The skin throws off about 16 ounces of toxic material daily in the form of perspiration—that is if your pores are not clogged with oils, lotions, and dead cells of yesteryears. It has been called the third kidney because of its ability to rid the body of toxic materials through perspiration and mucous secretions. Your body makes a new top layer of skin every 24 hours. Dry skin brushing removes the old, dead top layer of cells and increases cell renewal. It is a befriending gesture that improves overall detoxification of your body.

Befriending With Dry Skin Brushing

This will assist in detoxifying the body by stimulating the blood and lymphatic systems, which, in turn, will benefit your immune system. Using a long handled, *natural-bristled* brush, gently brush in small circular motions up your legs towards your belly, then to your hands, up your arms, and towards your chest. Do this for three to five minutes. Brush off the past and be open for the new. Invigorating, right? Benefits of dry skin brushing include:

▷ Opening of the pores, allowing your skin to breathe and toxins to be released.

▷ Stimulation of oil-producing glands (regular skin brushing can save you money on body creams and oils) and leaves skin fresh and glowing.

Note: Avoid brushing rashes, skin irritations, open wounds, and genitals.

Hydrotherapy: Healing With Water

When we stress-aholics think about giving ourselves a treat, a nice hot bubble bath or a trip to the steam room should be right up there with new shoes or a night out.

Hydrotherapy is the therapeutic use of water to treat physical and emotional disease and discomfort. Because of water's numerous physical properties and its comforting emotional associations, it has been used since the dawn of time as a powerful healing modality.

Using the combination of hot and cold water can be an extremely powerful modality to increase the circulation of nutrient-rich blood flow to the organs, to move out blockages of stagnation, and to enhance immune function. Healing naturally follows this process.

Cold water constricts blood vessels and moves stagnant blood and lymph fluid out of congested areas. It is beneficial in reducing inflammation. Cold is physically as well as emotionally invigorating. Hot water baths, sauna (dry heat), and steam (wet heat) stimulate toxins to be released from our cells into the lymph fluid, then out of our bodies through perspiration. Hot relaxes muscles and takes pressure off agitated nerves. Hot is emotionally and physically sedating—a natural tranquilizer, with no side effects. Some forms of hydrotherapy include hot/cold water flushes, saunas, steams, detox baths, enemas, and colon therapy. Experiment with any of these to assist you on your healing journey.

Befriending Invitation

Hot/Cold Flush: Start with a hot shower for two minutes, and then give yourself a blast of cold water for two minutes. Focus the water some of the time on your abdominal area. Repeat this cycle three times. End this exhilarating experience with a brisk towel rub. This process brings fresh blood and nutrients to tense areas (especially the gut), relieves cramping, and is a shot of natural energy.

Detox Baths, Saunas, Steam Rooms: These treatments raise the body temperature slightly, which increases metabolism and inhibits the growth of harmful viruses or bacteria. Slightly overheating your body encourages a slight fever-like response, an old traditional treatment for disease. A slight fever is the body's wisdom, generated by the immune system to "kill off" harmful microorganisms. Sauna, steam, and detox baths help you eliminate large amounts of toxins via the skin, your largest eliminative organ. This helps take the burden off your liver, kidney, colon, and lungs (your other eliminative organs).

Note: Saunas and steams should be avoided if you have high blood pressure, have very low blood pressure, or are pregnant.

Detox Baths

1. Begin by brushing off the past with dry skin brushing.
2. Add 1 cup of Epsom salts per 60 pounds of body weight to bath water as hot as you can comfortably tolerate. Epson salts contain magnesium, which relaxes muscles, and sulfur, which increases blood supply to the skin.
3. Soak for 20 minutes. (If you feel light-headed, please stop and get out of the tub.)
4. Do not use soaps, lotions, or oils. You want your skin to breathe and release toxins freely.
5. Shower in tepid/cool water.
6. Follow with a brisk towel rubdown to wipe off released toxins and enhance circulation.
7. Drink plenty of purified water to prevent dehydration.

Saunas and Steams

1. Begin by brushing off the past with dry skin brushing.
2. Whether you choose a sauna or steam, start off with 10 minutes and increase to 20 minutes as your tolerance allows.
3. Shower in tepid/cool water.
4. Follow with a brisk towel rubdown.
5. Drink plenty of purified water to prevent dehydration.

Colonics and Enemas

Put a hose where?! Shoot water up where?! Are you kidding?! No way, no how!

I've heard all of these responses a thousand times. Because of our culture's lack of understanding and general squeamishness surrounding our elimination functions, many don't realize the benefits of colon hydrotherapy. So let me give you a little insight into a healing process that has been around for thousands of years.

Colon hydrotherapy, in the form of an enema, was first used by ancient Egyptians in 1500 B.C. Hippocrates reported using enemas for treating fevers. The Essences (an ancient sect of holy men and women believed to have taught the seeds of Christianity) used such a process to rid the mind and spirit of the unclean and the body of disease.

In the early 1900s, J.H. Kellogg, M.D. (renowned for creating corn flakes), popularized colon hydrotherapy in the United States. In a 1917 issue of the *Journal of the American Medical Association,* Kellogg reported that he was able to assist all but 20 of his 40,000 patients in alleviating gastrointestinal illnesses without surgery, by using diet, exercise, and colon hydrotherapy (enemas). Truly the road back to Wellsville expressed! Kellogg's success with enemas inspired the development of the procedure known as colonics (aka colon therapy or colon hydrotherapy). Colonics are basically a more thorough and complete form of an enema.

In the early 1920s, colon therapy was used for the purpose of regaining health. "In 1920, colonic equipment was as common in doctors' offices as EKG machines are today. Colon therapy was mainstream medicine and a review of papers published at the time (all by medical doctors) confirmed the effectiveness of treatments in a wide variety of illnesses beyond the limits of the digestive tract," states D.D. Edelberg, M.D., clinical director of American WholeHealth Center, in his article, "Colon Therapy" in *Conscious Choice*.

Then, along came our fascination with and advancement of antibiotics, drugs, and surgery. Bowel purification practices seemed archaic, and we were taught to seek instant, immediate relief of symptoms and to often ignore the *root causes*. Colon therapy, after taking a backseat to so-called modern medicine for years, is enjoying a resurgence, mostly in holistic communities, especially because many are not getting relief from conventional medicine.

Presently, many progressive physicians are recommending colonics as an adjunct to their treatment regimens. In Dr. Morton Walker's article, "Value of Hydrotherapy Verified by Medical Professionals" (in the August/September 2000 edition of the *Townsend Letter for Doctors and Patients*), he interviewed doctors who were enthusiastically prescribing and/or using colon hydrotherapy as part of their treatment protocols for constipation, allergies, prostatic hyperplasia, cancer, and more.

Dr. Robert Charm, a board-certified gastroenterologist, prescribes colon hydrotherapy. He confides that when he performs a colonoscopy on many of his patients, their bowels are filled with pockets of waste matter:

"Some patients have held on to the stool pockets for decades. A toxic dumpsite like this is dangerous.... Environmental cancer can develop!" He also states that it is a safe technique that gives relief to IBS, constipation, and many other gastrointestinal problems.

Pamela Whitney, N.D., who prescribes colon hydrotherapy for many of her patients, states: "The patient's toxins tend to kick back to the blood stream to perpetuate numerous pathologies such as candidasis, allergies, chronic fatigue and other symptoms coming from a recirculation of accumulated physiological poisons....I don't know of any patient receiving colon hydrotherapy who has not benefited from it."

Colonics

Colonics are a gentle, internal bath for your colon. Unlike enemas, which only reach the lower (descending) portion of the lower intestine, colonics are able to reach all parts of the large intestine. They are not solely a treatment for constipation but are intended to rid the body of accumulated toxins from drug residue, candida die-off, gas, bacteria, food cravings, and autointoxification.

A person receiving a colonic lies on a table, where a *sterilized* speculum is gently inserted into the rectum. Water flow, which is always under the direct control of the trained practitioner, flows into the colon via a small tube. The individual is filled with a certain volume of water to his or her tolerance. This process will induce gentle colon-muscle contractions. The water then flows out via an evacuation tube, bringing with it wastes, gas, and mucous. As the water flows out of the colon, the practitioner gently massages the abdomen to help the colon release its contents. The procedure is completely professional, and modesty is given top priority. The colonic process takes only 20 to 50 minutes. Generally, a series of colonic treatments (six to 12) is recommended. Remember: It usually takes years of neglect for the colon to become congested with waste products. Patience, internal cleansing, and attitude and diet changes will bring positive results in a relatively brief period of time.

Conditions That Can Benefit From Colon Therapy?

▸ Constipation, IBS, gas, bloat, skin conditions, headaches, aches and pains, fatigue, candida, fever, and flu. (See "Autointoxication" in Chapter 3.)

▸ Para/quadriplegics. (Colon therapy assists in bowel training.)

▸ MS, lupus, cancer, ALS.*

▶ Detoxing system of alcohol and drugs.

▶ Preparation and post-barium X-ray.*

▶ Reduce the side effects of chemotherapy (such as nausea and poor appetite).*

▶ Preventive to colon cancer.

▶ During diet and lifestyle change.

▶ During a cleansing or fasting program to reduce detox symptoms.

▶ Physically or/and emotionally stuck.

*Used only with doctor's release.

Befriending Gifts of Colon Therapy

▶ **Detoxification.** Colon therapy clears the colon of potential toxic troublemakers as it coaxes your body to remove old stools, gases, accumulated mucous, and parasites. These toxins can contribute to symptoms such as bloat, headaches, muscular aches, allergies, nausea, fatigue, lower backaches, skin conditions, and a compromised immune system. Some of these toxins can be carcinogenic and can alter the structure of the cells, creating cancerous cells.

▶ **Exercises colon muscles.** Water aerobics for the gut! When waste is allowed to remain in the gut, the colon muscles weaken, thus leaving the gut like a 90-pound weakling, unable to function properly. The gentle process of filling and emptying with water improves the colon's peristaltic (muscular) movement, thus improving transit time and all-over colon function.

▶ **Stimulates colon reflex points.** Every system and organ in our body is connected by reflex points. Through the process of a colonic, the reflex points are stimulated, thereby affecting corresponding body organs, glands, tissues, and so forth. (See the diagram on page 136.)

▶ **Promotes body awareness.** Once the colon is cleaner, one becomes very aware of the effects of food and substances on the gut. For example, when you are bloated, gassy, and constipated, you generally have no idea which food or habit is causing which symptom. After you have a colonic, you have wiped the slate clean, so to speak. As you ingest a foe food, your gut wisdom will speak. You may immediately notice the bloat, gas, or cramping occurring, guiding you to the cause and effects of your food choices. Your food-gut relationship awareness heightens.

■ ■ ■ ■ ■ ■ ■ ■ ■

Reflex Points

The concept of reflexology, which states that there are reflex points in the feet, hands, and ears that correspond to various organs, glands, and areas in the body, is fairly well known. However, it is not generally understood that there are reflex points in the colon, as well.

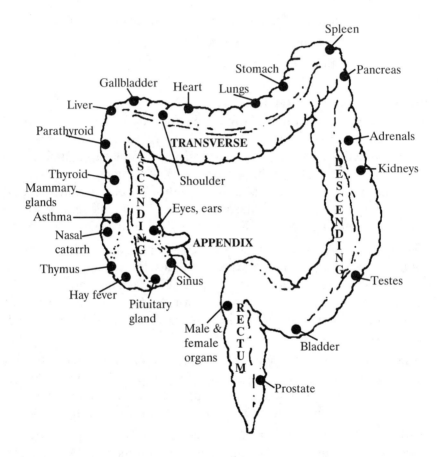

Adapted from *Colon Health*
by Norman Walker, D.Sc., p. 10

■ ■ ■

▶ **Emotional clearing.** Our transverse colon passes right through our solar plexus—our seat of emotions. If emotions are held, "undigested traumas" linger, and our solar plexus/transverse colon area may be tight and tense. A colonic can bring awareness as well as assist in releasing these "held" toxic emotions.

Edgar Cayce (1877–1945), a medical intuitive and advocate of "internal cleansing," stated: "I have come to learn that cleansing the colon helps to heal negative feelings and old emotional traumas, for water is spirit and bring light into the soul, as well as into dark areas of the colon."

▶ **Happy hormones.** Because the gut (brain) manufactures more serotonin than your cerebral brain, there is a possibility that serotonin may get released during a colonic, leaving an individual with a sense of calm and clarity.

▶ **Psychological.** Because many feel so "clean" after a colonic, they choose healthier foods for their guts and thus improve body and mood.

There are many roads to a healthy gut. Colon therapy is an extraordinarily powerful tool when used with the other gut-befriending gestures (diet, breathing, and so forth). Colon therapy is the quickest way I've seen to help relieve symptoms and *immediately* get the gut back on a healthy track. *Some* of the common benefits one can experience undergoing colon therapy are the relief of nausea, bloat, and gas, dissipation of muscle aches, and clearer skin and sinuses. You may also notice diminished food cravings, allergy relief, headache alleviation, and improved bowel function. (If you have a "gut feeling" that this is a procedure for you, check Appendix C for help in finding a certified colon therapist in your area.)

Testimonials

"I have struggled with IBS for seven years now. Since I have been getting colonics, I've almost forgotten I even have a problem. I have tried everything, and this is the *only* thing that's worked."

—Kellie H.

"I am an exercise addict, but the pouch in my belly never changed. After a series of colonics, it's gone! An extra benefit I received was that my skin is clearing up—hallelujah to colonics!"

—Jenny W.

"I am a chemotherapy patient. Days after each chemo treatment, I would feel extremely nauseous, fatigued, my bowels were always upset, I had very little appetite, and had an overwhelming feeling of hopelessness and despair. With permission from my oncologist, I began colon therapy treatments. Within the hour of my first treatment, my nausea was totally gone. I was less tired, my appetite slightly improved, and I felt hopeful. Thank you, thank you, thank you."

—Bridgette G.

"I've suffered with painful constipation since my teens. I am now 44 years old. My doctors told me it was 'normal,' to not worry about it and just eat fiber. After receiving colonics and adjusting my diet, I have had—for the first time in my life—*easy* bowel movements. Extra bonuses experienced from colonics are the vanishing PMS symptoms and nagging lower backaches. I want everyone I know to get colonics."

—Susan K.

Enemas

Enemas are a valuable tool in helping to release stuck, constipated bowels or as a part of a cleansing program. They are not as thorough as a colonic but, for at-home relief, they can accomplish a great deal. You'll need a 2-quart enema bag, a catheter extension tube with connector, a tube of water soluble lubricant, a towel to lie on, and an hour of private time. Here's the procedure:

1. Wash the catheter tube with soap and water and rinse well.

2. Fill the enema bag with warm water (ideally purified water). Hang the bag 3 feet from the floor, allowing the catheter to rest on a paper towel on the floor.

3. Open the clamp on the tubing and allow some water to flow through the catheter into the toilet to clear any air in the tube, then reclamp the tube.

4. Lie down and take a few deep breaths to relax your body.

5. Lubricate the end of the catheter tube.

6. Lying on your left side, insert the catheter tube.

7. Allow the water to flow in and massage the lower colon. After a minute or two, remove the catheter and release the water into the toilet to unblock the lower colon of solid wastes.

8. Insert the tube again allowing water to flow in. Gently massage up the left side of the colon. Try to hold the water 10 or 15 minutes. While holding the water, keep massaging on the left side of your lower abdomen. This helps to loosen waste and break up gas pockets.

9. Remove the tube. Evacuate.

Wisdom Squat

Little do many of us realize that the act of sitting on our toilets may inhibit our gut's optimum functioning. It's back to basics, which means: *squat*! Squatting is the natural position for moving the bowels. The squat tends to stretch open the anus while the thighs press into the lower abdomen area, aiding in an easier movement of waste from the colon. By putting a foot stool at the base of your toilet, and placing your feet upon it, you can simulate a squat. By adopting the squatting posture, we allow the bowel to resume its function as nature intended.

Is Your Toilet Your Enemy?

The fact that people suffer from incomplete elimination was verified by Dr. John Chiere. Convinced that the toilet was faulty in design, he actually weighed and compared his fecal mass passed on the toilet with that passed in a squatting position. (John, get a life!) He found that he always eliminated less while using the toilet.

The majority of bowel problems, even as severe as cancer, are often located in two areas of the bowel: the cecum (the lower right area) and the sigmoid (the lower left area). These are the two areas massaged, supported, and thereby stimulated by the thighs when you squat. When we sit normally (without a foot stool) we apply no mechanical pressure in these areas and often strain and bear down, which can often contribute to hemorrhoid development. The bowel kinks and allows fecal matter to accumulate there, thus inviting unfriendly bacteria to flourish. The accumulating bacteria contribute to gas, bloat, constipation, as well as other gut ailments. Listen to your gut—and befriend it with a foot stool and a squat.

Movement/Wisdom-cises

Flowing water never stagnates, active things never rust.
—Master Sun Mo Ssu, Chinese physician 700 A.D.

Calling all couch potatoes! Your gut is a happy camper when you incorporate a program of daily exercise and stretching. Movement is a prerequisite for maintaining the health of your body and gut. All of the muscles in your body respond well to exercise, and the muscles in your intestinal tract are no exception.

Our bodies were designed for movement. If you are a couch potato, so is your circulation (blood and lymph and energy systems). Your digestive and elimination systems follow suit. A lack of flexibility is associated with "energy blockages." You become physically and emotionally sluggish and fatigued. Stress remains stuck in your gut with repercussions we are all too familiar with. Anxiety, depression, and daily agitation are exacerbated, which, in turn, affects your ailing belly. Here are some benefits of movement:

> It strengthens and tones the muscles of your digestive tract and helps stimulate blocked energy and a stagnant, sluggish bowel.

> A regular aerobic exercise program helps reduce stress and improves your mood by releasing endorphins, those feel-good hormones. Voila! Good digestion accompanies this befriending gesture.

> Movement enhances the removal of toxins. With movement, your circulation and perspiration increase. Via your sweat and breath, you let go of toxins circulating in your bloodstream and lymphatic system.

> Movement transports oxygen and nutrients to your cells, which can result in a stronger immune system.

> Exercise and stretch with breathing; it helps all areas of the body and especially the large intestine and lungs. Stimulating these muscles will assist in toning and relaxing the colon.

> Because "stuck," unreleased emotions may manifest themselves as physical symptoms (the gut's wisdom) in the body and gut, you may also use movement as a tool to bring awareness to your "holding" or "stuck" places. Use movement as an opportunity to let go.

How do you begin? All movement is good—just do it. If you are a true "potato," begin befriending your gut with exercise in little steps. Use the stairs instead of the elevator. Find a scenic route and begin walking for 10 minutes a few times a week. Explore movements and exercises that are enjoyable for you.

If you are already an exerciser, great. Keep it up! These particular stretches and movements shift stuck, blocked, tight holding areas in your body and gut. They assist in strengthening, toning, and allowing nourishing blood to flow to previously blocked areas.

Befriending Wisdom-cises

Following is a series of gut wisdom-cises (gut-health stretches and movements) intended for both the couch potato as well as the avid exerciser.

- ▷ Breathe. Never hold your breath. Inhibited breathing contributes to holding, tightening, and restricting an already-blocked region.

- ▷ Notice where you are holding. The "held" area will possibly feel tight or uncomfortable. Notice it; breathe deeply. As the restricted area releases, you will be able to stretch and open up further.

- ▷ Do each exercise slowly and deliberately.

- ▷ Relax after each exercise in order to feel your new openness.

- ▷ Practice these exercises daily for greatest benefits.

The Bicycle

Lie on your back. Bring your legs up and support your back with your lower hands. With your legs slightly bent, begin peddling your legs as if you were riding a bike. Do this 15–20 times.

Squats

Stand with your feet squarely on the floor. Place your hand on hips. Slowly and deliberately lower yourself into a squatting position, and then slowly come back up to the original stance. If necessary, use a chair for balance. Remember to breathe. Repeat 25 times.

Cat Stretch

On all fours, let your head drop, inhale deeply, and arch your spine high. Pause. With a long exhalation, let your back drop back down until it "hangs" naturally. Breathe easily for a few moments. Repeat four times.

Forward Bend

Sit on a firm surface, with your head, neck, and back in a straight line. Put your legs together in front of your body with the back of your knees flat on the floor. Inhale as you stretch both arms over your head, reaching up alongside your ears. Exhale and slowly bend forward from the hips. Reach forward and grab hold of your feet as you bring your chest down toward your thighs. If you can't reach your feet, grasp your ankles, shins, or knees. Breathe deeply into where you feel tension. Hold this stretch for at least 10 seconds. Slowly release the stretch. Inhale and stretch your arms and body up. Lay back and relax.

Leg Folding

Lie on your back. Grasp your right knee with both hands and bring it up gently against your chest (or close to it). Slowly inhale and exhale while lifting your head so that your forehead rests against your knee. Hold this position for three to 10 seconds. Release; then repeat with your left knee. Repeat this sequence up to five times.

Castor Oil Pack

Your nose may have just turned up with memories of Mom giving you a teaspoon of castor oil to help "get things moving down there." Internally, castor oil can be a gut irritant.

Well, this is not about an oral ingestion but a healing *topical* application of the old standby. It was used by the Egyptians 4,000 years ago, as well as by the ancient Greeks and ancient Indians. Castor oil was given the name Palm Christi (Palm of Christ) in the Middle Ages because of its great healing abilities. Castor oil's place in modern healing was often recommended by medical intuitive Edgar Cayce and was popularized by one of his disciples, William McGarey, M.D. Dr. McGarey directs the Association for Research and Enlightenment (ARE) Clinic in Phoenix, Arizona. Castor oil was and is presently used for many types of ailments, including conditions involving lymph flow, adhesions, inflammation, constipation, IBS, gastritis, colitis, and gall bladder and liver disorders.

Befriending Castor Oil Packs

Benefits of castor oil include:

> ⮞ It increases the movement of lymphatic fluid, which in turn enriches the immune system. The lymphatic system plays a key role in the absorption and assimilation of foods and acts as a cleansing or drainage system for cellular wastes.

> ‣ It assists in reducing gut tenderness and inflammation in conditions such as colitis, IBS, gastritis, and constipation.

Befriending Process

What you will need: 100-percent pure, cold-pressed castor oil, a plain wool flannel cloth large enough to fit over the entire abdominal area, a bath towel, a plastic sheet (Saran wrap or a plastic bag will do), and a heating pad, hot water bottle, or Belly Buddy.

Saturate the flannel with castor oil. Place the saturated flannel onto the abdomen. Cover your abdomen with the plastic and then with a towel. Apply your heating pad over the pack. Leave in place for one hour. It is recommended that the castor oil pack be applied for at least three consecutive days.

While using the castor oil pack, relax, belly breathe, and be aware of thoughts, feelings, sensations, and images that may arise from your inner wisdom. Be open, curious, and gentle with all that surfaces.

When you have finished, wash the oil from your abdomen with a pint of warm water to which you have added a teaspoon of baking soda. You can keep the oil-soaked flannel sealed in a sealed plastic bag or a jar. It is reusable as long as the oil doesn't become rancid or the flannel doesn't become discolored. Castor oil will stain linens, so be careful (or use older linens).

Wisdom Journaling

Journaling is a private way to get all those negative thoughts and irritations *out*. It is an awareness process to see and hear many of your thoughts and beliefs that are gut-stress inducers—and that no longer serve you. Journaling is a powerful way to connect with, get in touch with, and cleanse out of your gut what you have been holding on to emotionally but don't have a safe space to vent or express.

Befriending gesture: Write uncensored for 15 minutes, allowing yourself an emotional and mental purge. Don't edit; let it rip! Discharge blocked energy, repetitive mental chatter, and obsessive toxic thoughts and feelings. Allow the hurts, angers, doubts, grievances, and sadness to pour out. Set yourself free. Get to know what lurks deep within. Don't judge or criticize yourself for the "toxic" stuff that may emerge. What you are doing is clearing a space for love, joy, life, and a well-functioning gut.

Forgiveness

Holding on to anger is like grasping a hot coal with the intent on throwing it at someone else—you are the one who gets burned.

—Buddha

What things have happened to you that you cannot forgive? Take a peek inside: Who or what gives your gut an uncomfortable knot or a flash of nausea? To forgive is to release the mind, heart, and gut—the repository of emotions—from past hurts and to cease resentment towards another or towards ourselves. We usually think of forgiveness in terms of other people, but sometimes what we really need to do is forgive ourselves. In either case, we often spend a lot of time and energy holding on to blame and guilt but not enough time forgiving. Forgiveness enables us to overcome feelings and attitudes of anger, resentment, despair, judgment, and helplessness.

These toxic feelings and attitude are a stress within our gut and may manifest as irritable bowel flare-up, gas, pain, bloat, constipation, nausea, or a serious illness. As stated earlier in this book, negative emotions suppress the immune response for up to 6 hours following just thinking about a negative emotional experience.

Dr. Bernie Siegal of the Yale University Cancer Society, author of *Love, Medicine and Miracles,* states, "Learning to let go of negative emotions is the key to healing." Dr. Siegal invites cancer patients "to see the illness as a message to redirect his or her life...to resolve conflicts with others, express anger and resentment and other negative emotions they have boiling up inside, to begin looking out for their own needs. And in doing so, the immune system becomes stimulated and healing takes place."

When we forgive, the body ceases to release harmful gut- and body-destroying stress hormones. The immune system is stabilized and strengthened. If you are feeling love, appreciation, gratitude, and forgiveness, every cell in your body responds to that emotion. So, it's time to forgive and let go, at least for your gut's sake.

To assist befriending your gut toward forgiveness, try the following simple, but powerful, ceremony:

Forgiveness Ceremony

What you will need:

> ⊳ A quiet space.
>
> ⊳ A bowl.
>
> ⊳ Paper and a pencil.
>
> ⊳ Matches.

1. Ask yourself: What or who do you chose to forgive so that you and your gut may be free to live fully, without pain and discomfort?

2. Take three belly breaths. Allow an event that needs your forgiveness to surface. Write from your gut—do not sensor yourself. Your gut's wisdom will guide you: "I, _____ (your name), choose to forgive and release _____ (who or what)."

3. Take a belly breath. Read what you have written aloud; notice where you feel it in your body/belly. What sensations accompany your "who or what"?

4. When you are ready, read the paper aloud, light the paper, place it in the bowl, and add, "I am now free from this disease. Amen! Hallelujah! It is so!"

5. Take a belly breath. Notice if any sensations in your belly/body have shifted or not. Just notice.

6. Thank yourself for having the courage and wisdom to let go.

This forgiveness ceremony can be done multiple times to continue releasing, freeing yourself from the past, and opening up to living in the present. This frees up previously bound-up energy for your healing journey.

> *Letting go: The wisdom of the ages teaches us that there is a time to hold on and a time to let go. There are cycles of meetings as well as partings. Life is about change, movement, and flow. Let go, forgive, and open up a space for The New.*
>
> —Unknown

Embracing the Discomfort and Conversations With Gut

*What is split off, not felt, remains the same. When it is felt
it changes.*

—Eugene Gendline, *Focusing*

How can a gut discomfort be turned into a wise, inner friend? How
can you use your Gut Wisdom to tap into your own healing abilities?

We usually have some disdain for our bloat and gut discomforts, and
we want them to go away—yesterday. Here are some ways you may have
treated your gut discomforts:

> ⟩   Avoidance or denial. You may have avoided discomforts by
> continuing to eat foe foods or by keeping busy with meaningless,
> frantic activity. This can be likened to ignoring a friend in pain
> and this often causes your gut to "cry" louder.

> ⟩   Struggle or resisting. Remember the saying *what we resist,
> persists*? Struggling or resisting through negative thoughts such
> as "I hate this bloat" and "I wish I could just cut this pain out of
> me!" often intensify the discomfort. Anger and frustration
> encourage abdominal muscle tension and the release of stress
> hormones that perpetuates a vicious cycle of gut distress. This
> can be likened to screaming at a friend in pain.

Many of us have responded in one or both of these ways, and we may
have recognized they haven't worked. Be open to experimenting with a
new way of being with your gut's wisdom. Make a new choice. What if you
were to *embrace* your symptoms or discomfort as a friend that embodies
a source of wisdom and insight?

Having conversations with gut is a way of embracing a process that
encourages awareness and relief of your discomfort(s) in a very focused
way. Your gut needs to be cared for, protected, listened to, and not judged
or ignored. Embracing conversations with gut brings surprising insights,
physical and emotional relief, and a shift in the way you view your symptoms (your gut's wisdom).

Discomfort is your messenger. It is attempting to let you know it needs
something: emotional healing from loss, betrayals, loneliness, hurtful situations; needing to place attention on food choices; needing to change a
stressful lifestyle. How can you get upset with that kind of information? If
you perceived this part of you as if it was a child in distress with needs that
must be attended to, then pushing it away or disliking it would probably
not put a halt to the cries, whines, screams, and pleadings.

Instead of ignoring your gut's discomfort, embrace and listen to it. Embracing your gut by bringing it comfort and compassion, listening, dialoguing, and showing gratitude for its guidance and wisdom is a gentle yet powerful way to get relief.

Yes, this may seem odd or difficult at first, but why not explore the opportunity of experiencing something new? Open up your curious and willing side and experiment with this process. You may be pleasantly surprised.

The Process of Embracing

As you embrace your gut's discomfort, try to focus on physical sensations rather than emotions. For example: *Fear* is a *feeling*; the butterflies or a knot in your stomach is the *sensation*. Working with the guts' physical sensation will make it easier for you to focus. As a gut sensation changes, your emotions and thoughts may begin to alter likewise.

Let's begin this befriending process:

1. Sit or lay down in a comfortable position.

2. Close your eyes to shut out distractions.

3. Take three deep belly breaths and bring your awareness to your gut.

4. Notice any sensation in your gut or surrounding body parts. Just notice—no need to do anything.

5. Take three slower, deliberate belly breaths.

6. Notice what sensation you feel in your gut. Pain? Numbness? Tightness? Hot? Cold? Knots? Butterflies? Fullness? Nausea? It's okay if you don't feel any physical sensations; just stay focused on your gut.

7. Once you identify a sensation, visualize a warm comforting blanket, nurturing hands, or a healing spiritual deity (God, "The Light," Buddha, and so on) that feels safe and nurturing to you. Feel that the source of comfort is surrounding your gut sensation, embracing it. How does that feel?

8. *Embrace* the sensations within your gut with the intention of acknowledging, supporting, and nurturing it, rather than changing it. Allow your discomfort to be embraced for as long as you feel guided.

9. Has your sensation changed, shifted, or disappeared? Continue this process with conversations with the gut.

Conversations With Gut

For years, Susan suffered from a diagnosed case of candida, a chronic yeast infection, as well as a bloated abdomen with recurrent constipation. She was meticulous about diet, supplements, and a cleansing regimen, but she experienced only moderate relief. I invited her to do the process of embracing and dialoging with her chronic discomfort: Conversations With Gut!

Embracing her discomforts and conversations with her gut got her in touch with her repressed (and sometimes not so repressed) anger she had toward her husband. She got in touch with how she didn't feel "safe" expressing to an overbearing man. The chronic candida kept her at bay sexually with her husband. Once she was aware of how she was using her body as an armor of protection, instead of her voice—her power—the light bulb went on! She enrolled herself in assertiveness classes and couples counseling. Three months later her candida condition and other gut voices (symptoms) had cleared up significantly.

Not every case of gut disturbance has a hidden emotional issue sitting beneath it, but a surprising many do. So, how do you discover what appears to be hidden within? Allowing yourself to have a compassionate conversation with your gut is a magical way in. Remember that the gut's brain takes in information, learns, and remembers. Conversations with gut is a process to access direct contact and guidance from your gut's brain. It's a process of asking and listening—then asking again and listening again.

Through this process, you allow your gut to speak to you through your thoughts, emotions, images, or sensations.

You may receive an intuitive thought and/or feeling about a situation that needs changing, expressing, and letting go, or maybe an anger or disappointment hidden within that needs healing may surface. Guidance on what to eat or not to eat may be sent to you. You may hear or feel the voice of your inner child, asking you to pay attention to it. Listen. Don't edit any responses that occur; trust it. You may want to try to write down what you see and hear, feel, and intuit. Keep a journal each time you converse with your gut in order to get "the message" that's being conveyed to you. Are you ready for a chat?

■　■　■　■　■　■　■　■　■

The Process of Conversations With Gut

1. Sit or lay down in a comfortable position.

2. Close your eyes to eliminate outside distractions.

3. Take three deep belly breaths and bring your awareness to your gut.

4. Ask the following questions as if you were speaking to a scared or wounded child. Ask, "I'm sorry you are not feeling good, why are you in pain?" Listen for a response. "What do you need now?" Listen. "What is the next step in helping us heal?" Listen. When you feel complete with this process, let your gut know that you'll be back.

5. Thank your gut's wisdom for this time you spent together. A thoughtful, befriending gift to give your gut is to place warmth on it so that it continues to feel connected, nurtured, and comforted.

6. You may have received profound insights during this process, or you may not have noticed anything. Do not be discouraged. Continue this embracing and communication process as often as possible. Remember that you are attempting to build a healthy relationship with your gut, and, as with any good relationship, patience and consistency are imperative.

■　■　■

You have learned the many befriending gifts you can offer your gut to soothe it, nurture it, and assist it back into working order. But one of the most transformational, befriending gestures to bring an ailing belly back to health is to wipe the slate clean, so to speak. The next chapter will show you how to do exactly that.

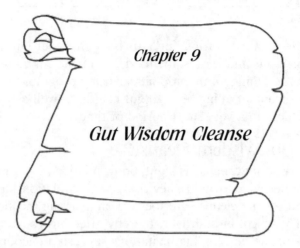

Chapter 9

Gut Wisdom Cleanse

*And the day came when the risk to remain tight in the bud
was more painful than the risk it took to bloom.*

—Anais Nin

I feel like somebody's old attic, stuffed with all kinds of garbage that nobody wants. There are old hurts here, old angers there, and leftovers from last Thanksgiving dinner! All this trash piles up until I can't function anymore. Won't you take out the garbage?

—Your Gut

Cynthia came to me complaining of chronic diarrhea, acne, yeast infections, and fatigue. The 31-year-old beautician was tired of her "work-hard, play-harder" lifestyle and wanted to learn to take better care of herself. The fried appetizers, beer, cigarettes, and hamburgers had taken their toll, and she was ready for a change. She opted for a seven-day Wisdom Cleanse. "At first," she said, "I was hungry. But then I realized that I had been using food as a reward." Throughout the week, she was sleeping better, she had clearer skin, she was experiencing solid bowel movements, and she'd dropped some weight. When she went back to her "normal" diet, she found that her body reacted strongly to the foe foods she'd always fed it and decided to stick with a healthier eating plan. Today, she is 10 pounds lighter and free of her chronic diarrhea. "Every day," she said, "I wake up more motivated. I have much more energy, and I'm actually craving vegetables."

One of the greatest befriending gifts is to give your gut a "vacation" from all the irritants and wastes, foe foods, and toxic emotions with a *Gut Wisdom Cleanse.* Doing an intentional cleansing program for 3 to 7 days can move you from an ailing belly to gut health, as well as correct other health imbalances in a very short period of time.

What Is a Gut Wisdom Cleanse?

The Gut Wisdom Cleanse is a gut, body, mind, and spiritual detoxification process designed to build a healthy gut-brain relationship. The products suggested for the cleanse are focused on assisting the cleansing and rebuilding of your colon and liver, thereby affecting your entire body's health. Some of the befriending invitations suggested encourage the letting go of physical, mental, and emotional blocks. Other invitations are designed to nurture, nourish, and replenish. Our body's wisdom knows how to heal. Our responsibility is to move the blocks out of the way and gently allow the healing process to occur. You are about to embark on a transformational process that has been used for centuries.

Since the dawn of time, fasting (abstaining from foods), enemas (they used hollowed out gourds in those days—ouch!), water, and herbs have been used as cleansing protocols. Spiritual leaders such as Jesus, Moses, and Krishna preached the wonders of cleansing for clarity of the mind, body, and spirit. Native Americans used cleansing as part of their spiritual practice to purify the body as a living temple of God. The Chinese would and still do use herbs for preventative healthcare. Currently throughout the world, health clinics and health-oriented spas implement various cleanses and fasts, thus successfully treating individuals from weight loss to cancer.

Why Cleanse?

The walls of our colon can become coated with layers of hardened waste and rubbery mucus from years of improper eating of refined, fiberless sugary foods. Many of us have overeaten to suppress or comfort ourselves during emotional times of frustration, loneliness, anger, and so forth. Medications have altered our gut's vital bacteria balance, causing irritated stomach and intestinal wall linings. Environmental toxins (pesticides, preservatives, pollution) have burdened our bodies with hazardous waste material. Stress has tightened our gut into knots and spasms as well as left behind degenerative chemical waste from the release of the stress-fighting hormones.

This literally creates a toxic waste site within us! Recirculating toxins (remember: What is not eliminated is recirculated) can overtax our liver and, consequently, other organs. This can contribute to various autoimmune dysfunctions as well as a myriad of other physical and emotional imbalances (see "Autotoxification" in Chapter 3).

Our body's wisdom does its best to protect us from these toxins by surrounding them with mucus, water, and fat. Toxins will remain in our body tissue and organs until they are *removed*. The Gut Wisdom Cleanse is the *mover*. When the constant, steady flow of foe foods into our body is interrupted for a brief period of time, a major shift in our biochemical process occurs. The release of toxins that are stored in the fatty tissue of our body can be eliminated. Buried emotions may "come out of the closet" to be felt and released. Mentally we can detox non-health-giving thoughts. Spiritually, blocks may be moved to open us up to a deeper connection— with our loved ones, with our self, with our God.

The Gut Wisdom Cleanse can assist you in the following ways:

> Move from gut distress to gut healing in a *very* short period of time.

> Relieve various symptoms body-wide.

> Let go of toxic attitudes, emotions, relationships.

> Assist you in identifying effects of foe foods and habits.

> Neutralize food and substance cravings.

> Rid your body of aches and pains.

> Recharge your energy.

> Open you up to receive all kinds of "nourishment."

> Clear your skin.

> Eliminate bloat and gas.

> Support weight loss.

> Still your mind and turn awareness inward for guidance.

> Open yourself up to a higher source or spiritual power.

> Physical, emotional, mental, and spiritual clarity!

■ ■ ■ ■ ■ ■ ■ ■ ■

Do You Need a Physical Cleanse?

❑ Do you suffer from digestive and eliminative distress?

❑ Are you overweight?

❑ Are you and your gut craving sweets and carbs?

❑ Do you get bloated after meals?

❑ Do you experience gas, belching, and heartburn?

❑ Is your skin blemished or sallow?

❑ Do you experience constant headaches or migraines?

❑ Are you vulnerable to sickness, frequent allergies, colds, sore throats?

❑ Do you suffer from constipation, IBS, candida, nausea?

❑ Are you tired even though you're getting enough sleep?

❑ Do you experience aches and pains? Arthritis?

❑ Do you have painful menstrual periods?

❑ Do you have difficulty thinking and concentrating?

❑ Do you have dark circles under your eyes?

❑ Do you have sinus problems?

❑ Do you have genital itch or discharge?

❑ Are you stressed out?

Do You Need an Emotional Cleanse?

❑ Do you eat when lonely, upset, and bored?

❑ Are you depressed often?

❑ Do you tend to hold onto old hurts, regrets, or grudges? Do you marinate in self-pity?

❑ Do you find it difficult to express emotions such as fear, anger, rage, grief, joy, love, or sexual feelings?

❑ Are you anxious, irritable, or quick to get angry?

❑ Does your mind constantly chatter negative thoughts or criticisms about yourself or others?

❑ Do you feel disconnected from your needs and desires, from other people, from your God, or from your sense of purpose?

❑ Can you be alone without constant distractions (TV, radio, telephone, books) and still be at peace?

❑ Do you feel stuck?

❑ Are you stressed out?

If you answered yes to five or more of any of these questions, then it's time for the Gut Wisdom Cleanse.

■ ■ ■

Wisdom Cleanse Testimonials

"I suffered from IBS for more than 15 years, and my stomach was always feeling upset. I think that I've tried just about every product and doctors in both the conventional and alternative methods. To my amazement, after the Gut Wisdom 3-day cleanse, I felt like I took a valium for my intestinal tract. I also lost six pounds and learned to 'treat my gut kinder' or as Alyce would say, 'befriend my belly.'"

—Heather M.

"I've embarked on many cleanses in my 55 years. I found the Gut Wisdom Cleanse exceptionally easy to finish. I opted for the seven-day Gut Wisdom Cleanse and had an interesting 'journey.'... I used chewing tobacco for four years and just quit a year ago. During the cleanse, my tongue turned black—whoa! I've experienced many things during my cleanse, but never this. By the end of my cleanse, my tongue cleared up. I can't help but feel this process of cleansing helped prevent a serious health condition in my future."

—Don H.

"I got clear on how 'toxic' my job was to me, how I used food to medicate my unhappiness and feelings of stuckness. After the cleanse I left my job of 15 years and was miraculously offered a new job in which I feel appreciated both verbally and financially. I listen to my 'gut feelings' and instincts now with new admiration and deep appreciation."

—Sabrina V.

■　■　■　■　■　■　■　■　■

"Let go and make room for what's new and what's next.
Let go and enjoy the excitement of not knowing what's next.
Let go and open up to all possibilities.
Let go when its time to yield.
Let go, and by doing so, gain freedom.
Let go and surrender to greater peace of mind."

—Marie Arapakis, Sufi Power Solutions

■　■　■

The Cleansing Journey

1. **Prepare to Let Go.** Most of the foods and substances we ingest are attached to an emotional component. During the cleanse, you will not be physically hungry. What might surface is emotional hunger. You may ask yourself what you are really hungry for. We eat and drink to repress, to comfort, to avoid, to reward ourselves. So in letting go, and moving these substances out of our way, there may be a surfacing of what has been "stuffed" down. Keep in mind to the best of your ability that this experiment of letting go is for the intent of a healthier relationship with your gut. What is your intention for this cleanse? Physical? Emotional? Spiritual?

2. **Do Your Personal Best.** Everyone is at different stages of personal growth, so take the program one step at a time. You might be a fast-food junkie whose decision to add daily vegetables may be a big step. Or maybe you are a health enthusiast and seek a refresher course on how to edit out certain types of foods and emotional holdings. What matters is a clear intention and to be gentle with yourself. *Remember that every step is a step toward your gut's health.*

3. **Be Gentle With Your Self.** If you find your car turning into the local McDonald's during your program, it doesn't mean you have to quit. Just pick up where you left off. Because food is such an emotional nourisher, medicator, and repressor, letting go of certain patterns may give rise to emotional upheavals. This is a great opportunity to become *aware*, perhaps of "toxic" emotions that surface and desires to be moved out. You see, "cheating" or wanting to cheat can be a way to explore deeper emotional issues that may be contributing to your guts distress. So, stay *aware*.

4. **If You Experience Symptoms...** Sometimes feeling worse means you're feeling better! During the cleanse, you may experience some symptoms that indicate that your body is trying to heal itself. These symptoms are known as a Herxheimer Reaction and are often caused by the die off of harmful bacteria. Your symptoms will vary according to the present condition of your health and what your gut and organs are willing to let go. You may experience skin breakouts, bad breath and/or body odor, copious amounts of and foul-smelling waste and gas, headaches, and flu-like symptoms such as muscular aches and fatigue. You may experience emotional stirrings during which there might be waves of sadness, anger, and irritability. On the other hand, you may feel peaceful, calm, and energized, be able to sleep soundly,

and have pains and discomforts subside. Each time you cleanse, it will be a different experience. So rest, sleep, take it easy. Enemas or colonics, drinking water, Wisdom Journaling, Movement, Embracing the Discomfort, and Conversations with Gut will all ease the healing reactions. If possible, do not take anything—aspirins, cold/flu medication, and so on—to suppress your symptoms. You want this "stuff" out. Vamoose, bon voyage, say goodbye! Be grateful to these symptoms, for it means the wisdom of your gut (body) is doing what inherently it knows how to do: *heal! We just need to get out of its way!*

Wisdom Invitations to Assist Your Cleanse

▸ **Intention.** Having a clear intention as to why you are cleansing will help keep you on track and make this journey purposeful. What would you like to let go of?

   ▹ Physically: muscle pain, bloat, constipation, headaches, or excess weight.

   ▹ Emotionally: anger, irritation, resentment, or self-pity.

   ▹ Spiritually: feeling disconnected from your source (your spirit, your God, your inner wisdom).

▸ **Let Go.** A week prior to the cleanse, begin letting go of your foe foods (sugars, refined flour products, alcohol, dairy, caffeine). Are you ready for a gut-brain transformation? What has been your "payoff" for your discomfort? What have you been holding on to that no longer serves you? Are you willing to let go? (Review "So the Gut Is the Messenger. What's the Message?" in Chapter 4.)

▸ **Colon Therapy.** During the seven-day cleanse, colonics are recommended on the first, third, and last days of the cleanse. For a three-day cleanse, two colonics are recommended. If you choose not to have a colonic, I encourage you to give yourself enemas. This process helps move out waste as well as reduces symptoms experienced by cleansing.

▸ **Castor Oil Packs.** These will assist in detoxifying toxins from your liver and gut. Three consecutive days is optimum.

▸ **Brush Away the Past.** Dry brush daily before you shower or bathe. This will remove dead skin and stimulate your lymphatic system to enhance the detoxification process.

▸ **Sauna/Steam or Detox Bath.** This should also be done daily to assist toxins out of your body.

▸ **Hot and Cold Flush.** This will stimulate blood and lymph flow.

▸ **Chew, Chew, Chew.** Digestion starts in your mouth. Support this amazing process by chewing your fruits and vegetables more and more until you can chew each bite between thirty and forty times. This will also help prevent excessive gas.

▸ **Movement.** Gentle exercise and gut stretching movements help stretch and stimulate your gut's function and assist in breaking up stagnation within the body.

▸ **Belly Breath.** Deep abdominal breathing releases toxins from your lungs, oxygenates your blood, and allows you to feel and release. Deep breathing massages your gut's organs, thus restoring proper function.

▸ **Belly Massage.** Massaging your abdomen helps move out stuck gas and waste. Notice feelings opening up and shifting as you massage.

▸ **Warmth on the Abdomen.** This calms and helps restore proper gut function. Warmth can be comforting and soothing and allow vulnerable feelings to surface.

▸ **Embrace the Discomfort and Conversation With Gut.** This is highly recommended during your cleanse. Progressively, you will be able to hear your gut's wisdom much more clearly.

▸ **Forgiveness Ceremony.** This is a powerful transformational process to do as you are cleansing and letting go.

▸ **Journal.** Writing is a great tool to get toxic thoughts and feelings out of you in order to support your healing journey. Move it out of you.

▸ **Rest.** Listen to your body. Rest. Cut back on activities. Allow your body to go through the many stages of letting go and getting healthy.

▸ **Read Inspirational Material.** Fill your gut, mind, and spirit with inspiring nourishment.

▸ **Reduce "Disconnectors" (TV, overwork, and so on).** This is the time to befriend and connect with your gut's wisdom. You are building a healthy relationship, so listen. Slow down and be aware of your feelings, attitudes, and physical symptoms. Be excited and curious as you notice all what surfaces.

▸ **Ask for Support.** Ask friends and family to help you during this cleansing period. Ask family not to bring home your favorite food or tempt you with your favorite restaurant.

For Your Wisdom Cleanse, You Will Need:

(See Appendix C for where to order some of these specialized products.)

Lemons are needed for your lemon flush. A cup of hot water and 1/2 squeezed organic lemon. This beverage promotes bowel peristalsis and benefits bile formation, which helps regenerate and detoxify the liver.

BioCleanse is a vegetarian rice-based protein powder designed to provide the specific ingredients that assist the liver in the process of removing toxins—both environmental as well as the toxic breakdown by-products formed by our own body processes. Substantial vitamins, minerals, and amino acids are included in this very supportive product. BioCleanse meets the nutritional needs during the cleanse process. The protein supplied prevents muscle wasting—a concern when one is fasting. The balanced portions of protein, carbohydrates, and fats help keep blood sugar levels balanced and energy levels up.

Ground flax seed is high in fiber and helps increase the volume of the intestinal contents. This increase in volume exercises the walls of the colon and encourages peristaltic activity in the bowel, absorbs toxins from the bowel, regulates levels of colon bacteria, and acts as a soother to the digestive tract. It supplies you with omega-3 essential fatty acids that have been used to reduce inflammation. It is one of the richest sources of antioxidants called lignins. Lignin fibers have been found to lower levels of cholesterol and prevent the formation of gallstones. It binds with bile acids, removing them before they form stones into a substance called mammalian lignin that can inhibit the action of "bad" estrogen linked to breast cancers. It has a pleasant nutty taste.

Vitamin C helps keep the immune system strong. It accelerates healing and repair of the body's cells and tissues and helps counteract fermentation in the gut. In higher doses, vitamin C can be used as a natural laxative. Studies have shown that vitamin C increases the activity or the white blood cells involved in fighting infection.

Acidophilus and bifidus are friendly bacteria will create an environment in your gut that is inhospitable for the unfriendly, toxin-producing, disease-causing bacteria. Acidophilus has many other desirable effects, including facilitation of the digestive process, production of important nutrients within the intestines, and stimulation of the immune system. It also may reduce some of the gas that occurs during a cleansing regime. You will need to use a nondairy, refrigerated source.

Super Green tablets are the basic foundation of health. By restoring an alkaline balance, greens enhance immunity. They are high in fiber, which increases bowel transit time and improves the tone of a weakened bowel. Suggested types: alfalfa tablets, wheat grass, spirulina, kamut, or chlorophyll tablets.

Herbal bowel formula improves the tone of the bowel and help to move waste matter out of the bowel. Some of the wonderful ingredients include barberry root bark, fennel seed, goldenseal, lobelia, red raspberry leaves, and turkey rhubarb.

Fresh vegetable juices are both cleansing and rebuilding for the system, and they're an easy way to take absorbable, usable nutrients into the body. They can break down and flush out toxins rapidly. Optimally focus on the green vegetable for your juice. "Greener" juices are excellent for mucus-cleansing, and they alkalize the body to a balanced internal state. They can be made fresh at home from your own juicer or purchased from a health food store juice bar. Be creative and include any combination of two or more of spinach, parsley, celery, kale, broccoli, apple, carrot, and ginger.

Wheat grass is rich in chlorophyll. This is a grass grown from wheat berry seeds. It contains more than a hundred vitamins, minerals, and nutrients and is believed to contain a number of cancer-fighting agents and immune-boosting properties. It detoxifies and strengthens the system. Many juice bars offer wheat grass.

Green tea is a now popular Asian tea. It is believed that green tea neutralizes free radicals, which are carcinogenic. It is also considered to be an anti-cancer tea, particularly for cancers of the stomach, lungs, and skin.

Pau D'Arco tea is an herbal cleansing agent, is an antimicrobial agent, and is reputed to stop tumor growth.

Wisdom-Replenishing Broth

This broth is a tasty and nourishing source of minerals and electrolytes. Use this if you are experiencing hunger during the cleanse. It is also recommended if you are lacking energy or recovering from a health challenge.

1 bunch beets	4 red potatoes (skins on)
4 stalks of celery (tops on)	3 carrots
1/2 head cabbage	1/2 bunch parsley

Put all ingredients into a large soup pot with 1 1/2 quarts of water. Bring to a boil. Reduce heat, simmer for 30 minutes. Strain. You can season the broth with 1 teaspoon of miso or a tablespoon of Bragg's liquid amino acids. This recipe makes approximately 6 cups.

You may also want to have on hand:

> Natural fiber skin brush or loofah to "brush off the past."

> Epsom salts for detox baths.

> A blender.

> A vegetable juicer or access to a health food store that makes fresh juices.

> A quart of your favorite sugar-free juice to mix with your Wisdom Elixir (see page 162).

> A hot water bottle or Belly Buddy.

> Castor oil and a flannel to do a castor oil pack.

> An open mind and a willingness to let go, listen, and explore new state of wellness, and the desire for transformation.

During your cleanse, include:

> Wisdom Elixir products.

> An abundance of vegetables.

> Fresh vegetable juice.

> Fruits.

> Wisdom Broth.

> Pure water and herbal teas (at least a gallon per day).

Foods to avoid:

> Junk food.

> Fried food.

> Meats, poultry, fish.

> Dairy products.

> Eggs.

> Flour products (breads, pasta, etc.).

> Alcohol.

> Caffeine.

> Sodas.

> Sugar.

> Salt.

Now that you are mentally and physically prepared for the cleanse, you are ready to begin.

The Wisdom Cleanse
Upon Rising
Drink a Lemon Flush: a cup of warmed water with the juice of half a lemon. Follow with the Wisdom Elixir.

In a blender, mix:

    4 ounces unsweetened fruit juice
    4 ounces purified water
    1 scoop BioCleanse
    2 heaping tablespoons ground flax seed
    1/4 teaspoon vitamin C powder
    1/4 teaspoon of acidophilus and bifidus
        OR two capsules

Then follow your Wisdom Elixir with 8 ounces of water, two herbal bowel formula (LBC-Lax) capsules, and three Super Green tablets.

Follow with the breakfast regimen 30 minutes to an hour later.

Breakfast
Enjoy fruits! Include a variety of fruits that are in season: apples, blueberries, grapes, kiwi, nectarines, peaches, pears, bananas, oranges, and cherries. Eat melons by themselves (a food combining rule).

Thirty minutes to an hour prior to lunch, have a second serving of Wisdom Elixir, two herbal bowel formula (LBC-Lax) capsules, and three more Super Green tablets.

Lunch
Lunch may include fresh crispy salads, steamed, baked, or stir-fried vegetables, or Wisdom Broth. Include various types of leaf lettuce (excluding the nonnutritious iceberg lettuce), sprouts (alfalfa, sunflower, beans), spinach, carrots, celery, parsley, cucumber, cabbage, broccoli, and/or beets.

Note: Salad dressing is not recommended during the cleanse. It is best to consider using olive oil and a squeezed lemon. Add herbs or Bragg's mineral broth (found in your local health food stores) for a little extra flavor.

Thirty minutes to an hour prior to dinner have your third serving of Wisdom Elixir, one herbal bowel formula capsule, and three Super Green tablets.

Dinner

Your dinner is the same as lunch. Experiment with a variety of different vegetables so you do not to get bored.

Snacks

In between breakfast, lunch, and dinner, include 8 ounces of fresh vegetable juice, water, and herbal teas. Attempt to drink eight glasses of purified water daily. Enjoy the suggested herbal teas or try other decaffeinated teas. You can also add Wisdom Broth if you get hungry between meals. For added detoxification, include 2 ounces of fresh wheat grass a day. (You may want to have a couple of ounces of apple juice as a "chaser" until you get used to the "green" taste.)

What if...

▶ ...you have diarrhea? Cut back on herbal bowel formula and one serving of VitC in your Wisdom Elixir.

▶ ...you feel weak? Check to see whether you included plenty of vegetables in your cleanse. Eat your Wisdom Broth. Are you drinking at least eight glasses of water daily? Remember to rest; your body is healing and may need some long overdue rest.

▶ ...you are on prescription medications? Continue your medications and consult with your doctor for a second opinion.

Breaking the Cleanse

Care and awareness are needed during this part of the journey. Cleansing may have been fairly easy, but breaking the cleanse and the follow-up are just as important. Resuming a healthy, normal eating pattern after a cleanse may be more challenging than the cleanse itself. If you jump back into the old habits, previous symptoms may reoccur and be back in your face or gut. Bummer—after all that work!

I suggest that you take at least half of your total cleansing time to gradually move back into a regular diet—that is, if your cleanse lasted seven days, take at least three to gradually break the cleanse. As you gently break your cleanse and resume regular eating, understand that it is with intention of altering your "regular" diet, following with the Gut Wisdom Diet (Chapter 6) along with "Keeping the Afterglow" (the following section in this chapter), which will help assist your healing journey.

This is a wonderful time to really *listen to your gut.*Because cleansing has heightened your awareness, your gut is your personal biofeedback machine, sharing with you the cause and effect of the foods you select. If you choose an inappropriate food for your gut, it will speak to you immediately. Notice when you begin feeding yourself health-defeating thoughts; be aware of relationships and situations that nourish you and those that don't. You have been empowered to continue a healthy relationship with your gut's wisdom. Listen to those "gut feelings." Listen, listen, listen! Food sensitivities may be discovered as you begin incorporating them into your program. Keep a wisdom food journal so you don't step into the ever-so-common "Alzheimer's" reaction of forgetting how your gut spoke to you and how you felt. Your communication pathways have been cleared; therefore your ability to listen to your gut's wisdom is heightened. Emotions and mental attitudes also may be highlighted.

Keeping the Afterglow

▶ Begin your day with a lemon flush.

▶ Follow that with a variation of the Wisdom Elixir. Mix 4 ounces of unsweetened juice and 4 ounces of water with one scoop of rice protein powder (or egg white protein power or, for a continued "lite" cleansing, continue with the BioCleanse protein powder). Add vitamin C powder (1/4 tsp.), acidophilus and bifidus (1/4 tsp. or two capsules), ground flax seed (2 heaping Tbs.), and a teaspoon of essential fatty acid oil to continue to heal your gut. Follow with 8 ounces of purified water and four Super Green capsules.

▶ Slowly and mindfully reintroduce friendly grains and proteins.

▶ Continue with an abundance of vegetables, fruits, and fluids daily.

▶ Continue drinking fresh vegetable juices, and always drink at least eight glasses of purified water per day.

▶ Continue to experiment with wisdom food combining.

▶ Continue with one to three herbal bowel formula capsules per day if your bowels are a bit slow. Discontinue as your bowel movements normalize.

▶ With each meal, take a comprehensive digestive enzyme to ensure proper digestion, reduce gas and bloat, and support the elimination function.

▶ Listen to your gut. Don't abandon it now! You've just spent quality time connecting and building a healthy relationship.

▶ Follow the Gut Wisdom Diet (Chapter 6).

▶ Continue the journey with the befrienders:
  ▷ Breath.
  ▷ Warmth.
  ▷ Belly Massage.
  ▷ Hot/Cold Flush.
  ▷ Embracing Conversation With Gut.
  ▷ Forgiveness Ceremony.

▶ Keep on transforming. Do a one-day Gut Wisdom Cleanse monthly to keep on track. Biyearly, embark on a 3- or 7-day Wisdom Cleanse. Keep transformation alive and moving!

Befriending Condensed

This is a general summary of all I've shared with you. The following invitations can give you and your gut wisdom support to continue the focus on a functional gut relationship.

1. **Fluids.** If you don't get enough water, stool dehydrates and will not be eliminated in a timely manner. Dehydration is one of the major causes of constipation.
   ▷ Drink at least eight glasses of purified water daily, which your body needs to maintain a sound GI tract.
   ▷ Avoid liquids within half an hour before and after meals.
   ▷ Include herbal teas, diluted fruit juices, and vegetable juices in your diet.

2. **Fiber.** Fiber is your personal, intestinal broom. Without it, you can be assured of an unhappy gut. Remember: There is no fiber in meat, chicken, fish, egg, cheese, or refined and white-flour products. Include daily servings of vegetables, fruit, whole grains (gluten-free, if you're sensitive), and legumes/beans and supplement with ground flax seed to ensure sufficient fiber intake.

3. **Supplements.** To ensure the proper protection and functioning of your digestive and eliminative systems, include daily:
   ▷ Super Green tablets are a great source of fiber, healing, and cleansing chlorophyll, vitamins, and minerals. Take two to six tablets daily. Especially recommended if your veggie intake is insufficient.

- Acidophilus and bifidus are friendly bacteria that protect the gut from the unfriendly bacteria that create gas, inflammation, and irritation. Suggested: two capsules, three times daily.

- Ground flax seed is a wonderful source of fiber and gut-healing essential oils. Use 2 to 3 tablespoons mixed in juice or protein drinks or sprinkled on salads.

- Essential fatty acids (omega-3 and omega-6) will protect gut lining and enhance your metabolism.

- Digestive enzymes assist your gut in breaking down foods, thus enhancing absorption of valuable nutrients. They prevent gas, indigestion, and constipation and also support your eliminative process. Include them with each meal.

4. **Friendly Foods.**
   - Be aware of food choices. Nourishing choices bring you into a healthy relationship with your gut.

   - Eat friendly foods! For example, consume lots of green, leafy vegetables, fruits, whole grains, legumes/beans, and baked and broiled chicken, fish, turkey, and tofu.

   - Don't overeat! Your body can only handle so much. The rest turns to fat and toxins. Eat in moderation and stop eating before you feel stuffed. If you are "stuffing," ask yourself what feelings you may be trying to suppress. Journal about these feelings.

   - Eat organic foods as much as possible. Health food stores have a large selection of organic produce, dry goods, and free range animal products.

   - Experiment with letting go of foe foods and substances such as flour, sugar, dairy, alcohol, tobacco, soft drinks, and caffeine that are often gut troublemakers. Try one food category at a time. Make sure you replace foe foods with a friendlier substitute so you don't feel deprived. For one week, earnestly try to keep out gut troublemakers outlined in the previous chapters and notice if there are any changes. Journal about these changes. Remember: If any food is difficult or impossible to let go of, it may be your main troublemaker!

   - Combine foods wisely to prevent fermentation (gas/indigestion) from occurring. Poor digestion can manifest as indigestion, constipation, fatigue, and water retention.

▷ Chew, chew, chew your food. Digestion begins in your mouth.

▷ To keep yourself on track, give yourself some cheat days. If your gut normally has a challenging time with, say, flour products, stay off those products and substitute with other products. Then, allow yourself to have some "forbiddens" on the weekend. Do it with a smile and a blessing so as not to create negative chemical reactions in your gut. If you fall off the gut maintenance program for too long, get back on track with a one- to three-day Gut Wisdom Cleanse.

▷ Keep *gut troublemakers* out! Limit medications. Antibiotics, in particular, upset the balance of favorable intestinal flora, disrupting digestion and elimination and lowering resistance to disease.

▷ Avoid eating when you are upset or stressed, because your digestion and elimination are altered and inhibited under stressful conditions. If you must eat, apply warmth to your abdominal area to help bring back proper functioning. Use a hot water bottle or Belly Buddy.

5. **Move Your Body.**
   ▷ All movement stimulates peristaltic action, the gut's bowel function. Plus, movement is a great stress-reducer and helps you release those happy chemicals, endorphins. Incorporating even a 10-minute walk into your daily routine can often relieve constipation. Plenty of rest, alone time, and regular sensible exercise provide the mellow, supportive environment in which an improved diet and/or cleansing program can do its best work.

   ▷ Exercise, walk, run, swim, dance.

   ▷ Practice gut release stretches and exercises.

   ▷ Belly breathe. Deep breathing is a simple but powerful tool that releases toxins, massages internal organs, and reduces stress. Breathing deeply allows you to open up, feel, and begin to experience repressed emotions that make your gut "speak" with symptoms. Each deep inhalation and exhalation allows your diaphragm to give your intestines a long-needed massage that increases bowel function.

6. **Emotional Health.**

    ▹ Stress, long-held grievances, fear, anger, and frustration all affect your gut more than any foe food. Learn to reduce stress by belly breathing. Be willing to let go of toxic thoughts, feelings, and attitudes. If necessary, use the support of a qualified, trusted body-mind therapist, friend, or clergy member. Prayer or meditation is also important.

    ▹ What toxic experiences, feelings, and attitudes are you holding on to? In your journal, write out these "holdings." Get it all on paper: all the sadness, grief, "how dare he, how dare she!" Continue letting go of what or who is toxic in your life, respectfully and gently, from your newly awakened, empowered self. Let forgiveness be your goal.

    ▹ Again, only eat when you aren't feeling stressed. Peace and calm enhance the digestive process.

7. **Listen to Your Gut.**

    ▹ Listen to the symptoms that are your gut's wisdom, your messenger. Heed the warnings early and be proactive with changes.

    ▹ When Mother Nature calls, answer. When you don't heed the call, the impulse your body sends when you need to go gets weaker and weaker. This causes your system to hold onto excess waste, which not only becomes toxic but also distends or spasms your bowel and weakens the "call mechanism" even more.

8. **Spoil Your Gut.**

    ▹ Warm your belly. Warmth from a Belly Buddy or hot water bottle can relax tight muscles in your abdomen. Warmth can also increase blood flow to the area, bringing healing nutrients and restoring digestive/eliminative function. Plus, it feels good!

    ▹ Try belly massage. Besides feeling good, belly massages also helps relax your gut, move trapped gases out, and bring healing TLC to your gut.

    ▹ Wisdom squat. Put a foot stool at the base of your toilet and place your feet on it. This squatting position allows your bowel to resume its function as nature intended.

9. **Internal Cleanse.**
   ▷ Biyearly, seven-day Wisdom Cleanses and/or shorter one- to three-day cleanses help you get back on track. Many people do a one-day cleanse weekly, others do it monthly, and still others embark on a three-day wisdom cleanse on a monthly basis. Listen to your gut and you will know how often and when.

   ▷ The power of cleansing your system cannot be underestimated. It is a great preventative as well as curative process.

   ▷ Don't abandon your gut after your cleanse. Pay attention to food choices, thoughts, and attitudes.

10. **Gratitude.** Thank your gut for the guidance and wisdom it has given—and is giving—you. Perfection is not the goal, but awareness is. Befriend your inner wisdom and do the best you can, and rewards of a healthier gut will be yours.

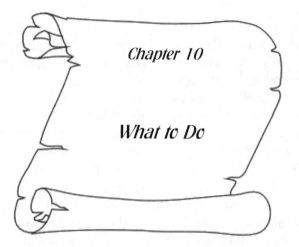

Chapter 10

What to Do

My barn having burned to the ground, I can now see the moon.
—Old Chinese Saying

Sometimes I need a little extra attention. A little natural vitamin here; a bit of an herb there; a dab of letting go of an old resentment works wonders. I'm not really needy; it's just that on occasion I work best when you focus on a specific discomfort in me—with natural remedies.

—Your Gut

Although modern medicine has made great strides in finding causes and cures for many of our gut ailments, we are still in the dark about the complexities of the human body—especially when it comes to coping with our gut issues.

On that note, I feel it's wise to say that we can't afford to ignore any methods that have been demonstrated in actual cases to be helpful in reducing or eliminating the sufferings of our guts. Drugs are a blessing and have their place in an emergency, but I believe there is no drug that doesn't have its penalty for prolonged use.

The application of herbs, diet changes, cleanses, breathing, movement, water therapies, and positive mental and emotional attitudes have been used for centuries with healing benefits and *no side effects*. As Hippocrates stated with his infinite gut wisdom, "Physician, do no harm."

A physician or your health practitioner cannot claim to heal you. All you and your physician or practitioner can do is to provide optimal conditions that will assist your gut in its natural healing process.

The wisdom of our gut offers us answers and clues to what is contributing to our gut's dysfunction, such as our improper food choices as well as our unhealthy attitudes. As we now know, each of these has biochemical and energetic effects within every cell of our bodies. The gut and brain function as an integrated whole. What we feel and think has an immediate effect on our physical body's health. What is experienced within our body undoubtedly affects our mental and emotional state.

As mentioned previously, the Chinese Taoists believed certain attitudes and emotions are correlated with specific ailments. Often there is a literal connection between our attitudes, the choice of emotional "nourishment" we take in, and the part of the body in which we experience the symptoms or discomfort. Symptoms are often attitudes manifesting physically. We think, "I can't stomach that person," and our stomach responds with nausea, constipation, or an irritable bowel flare-up.

Be open and explore all possibilities contributing to your gut's dysfunction, and allow your gut's wisdom to speak and offer its guidance. In this section, you will find a list of common digestive and eliminative ailments, along with possible contributors, from the foods you eat to the emotional and psychological attitudes and beliefs (gut-brain connections) you've ingested. The befriending invitations that are offered throughout the chapter can lead to improvement—sometimes moderate, sometimes miraculous. Choose three or four invitations you feel guided to, and work with them for two weeks. Listen, notice the changes; then add on two or three more. I cannot promise a cure, but I can assure you that, as you implement the befriending invitations, you will experience significant shifts to your gut health—all with the pleasant side effect of a gentle, comfortable bathroom experience.

Be open, willing, and curious. Look at all the possibilities of what may be contributing to your own ailing belly.

Constipation
What Is It?

You huff and you puff and still can't get it out. When your waste remains too long within you (ideal transit time is 18–24 hours), it becomes dry, hard, and difficult to release. Constipation results when waste material moves too slowly through the bowels, causing infrequent and often uncomfortable elimination.

Stagnant wastes become a cesspool, irritating the delicate lining of your colon and allowing toxins to be reabsorbed back into your bloodstream. This compromises the health of the rest of your body. Symptomatic conditions include headaches, skin conditions, fatigue, bad breath and body odor, coated tongue (a white coating on the tongue), and muscular aches, to name a few. Every organ and tissue is affected (see "Autointoxification" in Chapter 3).

Approximately eight million Americans suffer from the discomfort of constipation. In fact, according to the American Cancer Association, 20 million people use laxatives annually. Constipation can be a precursor to hemorrhoids, diverticulosis, diverticulitis, fatigue, headaches, depression, candida, and autointoxication. Constipation can be at the root of a majority of symptoms and disease—the "voice" of the gut.

Constipated stool not only moves slowly through the intestine, but it also deposits layer upon layer of slimy mucus on the walls of the intestine, where they gradually can become impacted and form tough, rubbery adhesions that obstruct the colon and thereby further delay elimination.

If constipation continues over a long period of time, your colon can get stretched or ballooned out or become narrow and contribute to spasms and abdominal aches and pains. The transverse portion of the colon can sag or prolapse, affecting your other organs. What you end up evacuating is skinny stool or round balls, rather than a full, fiber-filled, easy-to-pass bowel movement. (See Chapter 3.)

Although conventional opinion says that one bowel movement every couple of days is normal, I steadfastly disagree. The three meals you ate today should easily leave two or three times tomorrow. As a colon therapist, I see amazing amounts of accumulated waste matter leave individuals. As we clear the gut and make dietary, lifestyle, and attitude shifts, the *multiple* symptoms vanish and a normal and regular elimination is experienced for the first time.

Out with the old and in with the new is a must for gut and overall health to be restored.

Gut's Wisdom (Symptoms)

- Less than one bowel movement a day.
- Insufficient stool eliminated.
- Hard, compact stool.
- Chronic gas and bloated abdomen.
- Straining in order to move bowels.
- Hemorrhoids.
- Candida.
- Indigestion.
- Irritable bowel syndrome.
- Bad breath.
- Fatigue.
- Body odor.
- Headaches.
- Skin problems.
- Coated tongue.

Contributor to Gut Dysfunction: The Gut-Brain Connection

Chinese Taoist sages referred to the colon as the "controller of the drainage of dregs." A more succinct title, I believe, could be "gut-brain garbage collector." If we don't let go of emotional "old garbage," our gut is affected biochemically and energetically. Not only can we be physically constipated, but mentally and emotionally constipated—stuck.

As children we are told by society to hold back many of our true feelings so that we can be "socially correct." Big boys or girls don't cry. If you can't say anything nice, don't say anything at all. In order to be "correct" we don't express our anger, grief, or passions. We medicate ourselves with food and stuff our feelings down. We breathe shallowly so that we can hold back our discomfort. Soon we need a powerful laxative just to *let it out!* Unconsciously holding onto unexpressed emotions or toxic memories can also be a manifestation of a fear of letting go and trusting.

Holding on generally creates more toxic feelings that, in turn, can cause confusion, depression, obsession, and anxiety. This perpetuates a cycle of gut-brain constipation.

How do you let go? Do you hold onto the past? Are there people (including yourself) or experiences you need to let go of and forgive? Do you hold on with toxic anger, guilt, fear, or self-righteousness?

Gut-Brain Attitudes

- Fear.
- Feeling "stuck."
- Fear of "letting go."
- Holding on to the past.
- Unexpressed feelings.
- Holding on to old, no-longer-beneficial beliefs, emotions, or attitudes.
- Emotionally vulnerable—a need to protect/armor sensitive feelings.

Additional Contributors to Gut Dysfunction

▶ **A diet lacking in fiber and fluids and packed with foe foods** (fat, sugar, refined flour products, coffee, alcohol) are on the top of the list of causes of constipation.

▶ **Food sensitivities and allergies** can alter the bowel's function, especially wheat and dairy products.

▶ **Being a couch potato** makes us sluggish. Lack of exercise slows all parts of us down, including the bowel's movement.

▶ **Enzyme deficiencies** or poor food combining contribute to our food putrefying, contributing to slower transit time.

▶ **Stress.** During times of physical or emotional stress, blood is shunted away from the abdominal area, compromising digestion and elimination. Our breath is shallow and inhibited, and the gut doesn't get the gentle massage from our diaphragm to keep our bowels moving rhythmically and efficiently.

▶ **Laxatives** may be habit-forming, weakening the colon to the point that it may not be able to work without them. The nerve cells in the wall of the colon can be damaged by long-term habitual use. Often one might increase the number of laxatives taken daily until the gut shuts down totally with no movement at all (see "Getting Off Laxatives" on page 225).

▶ **Medications.** Painkillers, antidepressants, sleeping pills, and other prescription drugs, as well as iron supplements, antacids, and antibiotics, can contribute to constipation.

▶ **Hormones.** Many women may be aware that around their menstrual cycle or during pregnancy (more hormone shifts), constipation occurs. A low level of thyroid hormone is also a contributor to a slow, sluggish gut.

▶ **Structural damage.** Maybe an accident or just sleeping all twisted up on the wrong mattress has brought your spine out of alignment. If vertebrae are out of alignment, the gut can be affected.

▶ **Not listening to Mother Nature.** Your gut will speak only so many times. The longer stool remains in your colon, the more water is absorbed, the harder the stool gets, and the more difficult it is to pass.

▶ **Diseases** such as lupus, diabetes, Parkinson's, multiple sclerosis, or colon cancer can all affect the gut's function.

Befriending Invitations for Creating a Functional Gut

▶ **Increase fiber foods** (especially dark green, leafy vegetables), fruit, legumes, and whole grains (brown rice, millet, amaranth, quinoa).

▶ **Add extra fiber** such as ground flax seed or rice bran (two to three tablespoons mixed into water or juice or sprinkled on cereal, salads, or vegetables) daily (avoid wheat bran, which is sometimes harsh and irritating to the gut), or Metamucil* or psyllium husks* morning and evening.

*Make sure to drink sufficient water when taking these bulking fibers.

▸ **Super Green tablets**, which include alfalfa, wheat grass, and barley green, are rich in fiber and can be a gut saver if vegetables are difficult for you to include into your daily food intake. Begin with two tablets daily; eventually increase to six tablets. Your gut will let you know the appropriate dosage.

▸ **Acidophilus and bifidus** encourage peristalsis (bowel muscle movement) and protect the gut from invasion by harmful bacteria. Too little friendly bacteria contributes to constipation. Include two capsules, three times a day or 1/4 teaspoon of each in powder form, twice a day.

▸ **Digestive enzymes** with your meals assist the digestive process, encouraging complete digestion and efficient elimination. Use as directed with each meal.

▸ **Herbal colon combinations** are gentle and safe herbal laxatives that increase colon peristalsis. They are used to strengthen and tone the colon's function while you are making dietary and lifestyle changes. Herbs to include: cascara sagrada, turkey rhubarb root, barberry root bark. These herbal bowel supplements are gentle, safe, and natural laxatives that help to increase colon peristalsis. One to three capsules at bedtime is recommended, but your gut will let you know how many capsules to take by the number of bowel movements you experience.

▸ **Magnesium** assists your peristalsis (bowel muscle function) by proper relaxation of the muscles. It is suggested that you take 400 to 500 milligrams daily.

▸ **Increase the amount of water you drink,** but remember: not with meals, as that dilutes precious digestive enzymes. Drink at least eight glasses of purified water daily.

▸ **Omit or limit soda, coffee, and alcohol intake,** for they all have a dehydrating and irritating effect on your gut. Dehydration is a major contributor to constipation.

▸ **Experiment** with letting go of foe foods and replace with friendly foods. Omit only one food a week so you can notice the cause and effect and so it doesn't feel stressful and put you in deprivation mode. Remember to always fill the void with a friendly substitute. (See Chapter 5). I have witnessed that omitting wheat, dairy, sugar, and alcohol have a profound healing gut response. Follow the Gut Wisdom Diet suggestions in Chapter 6.

▸ **Eat when you are calm.** A stressed, irritated gut is a shut-down gut.

▶ **Chew, chew, chew.** Several studies conducted at major universities indicate that the enzymes in saliva continue their digestive activity in the upper stomach. Better digestion leads to better elimination and less gas!

▶ **Wisdom food combining** supports good digestion that, in turn, enhances proper elimination.

▶ **Omega-3 oils** such as flax, borage, and fish are effective in providing necessary lubrication for an easy and gentle elimination. Take one to three capsules daily.

▶ **Castor oil packs** assists proper liver function that, in turn, affects gut function. Use for three consecutive days.

▶ **Take deep belly breaths.** A deep abdominal breath gently massages and stimulates your colon plus reduces stress and enhances the restorative function of your nervous system.

▶ **Warmth on your belly** from a Belly Buddy or hot water bottle relaxes tight muscles in your abdomen and increases blood flow to your gut, bringing healing nutrients and restoring proper functioning. It invites comfort and nurturing, plus it feels good!

▶ **Belly massage** releases tight abdominal muscles and moves out stuck waste and trapped gas. This allows you to explore and release physical and emotional "holding" areas.

▶ **Exercise and wisdom-cises (stretches)** are gut releasers, and they keep your peristaltic action (gut's muscular movement) operating optimally.

▶ **Adjust your spine.** Visit a chiropractor, naprapath, or osteopath. If your lower back has been injured or vertebrae are out of alignment, this can put pressure on the spinal nerves that affect the health and movement of your gut.

▶ **Hot/cold flush** stimulates a stuck, stagnant, constipated gut. Do daily.

▶ **Comprehensive Digestive Stool Test** (CDSA) will check for candida, parasites, or other microorganisms affecting the function of your gut. Food allergy tests and/or thyroid tests are also suggested.

▶ **Listen and obey the call of Mother Nature.** When the urge is present, go. Otherwise dehydration can occur, contributing to dry, difficult-to-pass stools. Train your bowels by making the time each day to have bowel movements.

▶ **Wisdom squat**, the natural position for moving the bowels. By putting a foot stool at the base of your toilet, and placing your feet on it, you can simulate a squat.

▶ **Wisdom Cleanse.** A one-day or three-day cleanse monthly, or a seven-day cleanse biyearly, is suggested. To get your gut on track, listen and follow your gut's wisdom.

▶ **Colonics** will help cleanse out old waste, gas, and discomfort associated with constipation. A colonic will offer you the long-desired release. It can help you become aware of causes and effects of your foods and your emotional holdings. Colonics are excellent to do in tandem with the Wisdom Cleanse.

▶ **A forgiveness ceremony** can help you let go of old emotions, feelings, beliefs, and attitudes that no longer serve you. Ask yourself, "What am I holding on to that no longer supports my emotional and physical health? Am I willing to trust and let go?"

▶ **Embracing your discomfort and conversing with your gut** can aid in discovering what is emotionally and physically keeping you "stuck."

▶ **Thank your gut** for its message of reminding you to let go and open up and trust what is new and nourishing.

Candida Albicans
What Is It?

Candida albicans is a yeast-like, parasitic organism found in each and every one of us—in our intestines, genital tract, mouth, and throat. This critter normally lives a quiet life in our mucous membranes, kept in check by our immune system and friendly bacteria. But, as you now know, your immune system can be compromised and friendly bacteria can be destroyed by your lifestyle: alcohol, sugar (a delicious way to feed yeast!), stress, antibiotics, and other medications.

When the bacteria that normally keeps candida in control are destroyed, it allows the candida yeast to multiply and flourish. When candida takes over the gut neighborhood, so to speak, our gut lining may become irritated. With long-term infestation, the yeast shifts into a fungus form where it develops "roots" that can implant themselves into the intestinal wall, causing small tears or leaks (this is called leaky-gut syndrome). A leaky gut is an intestinal lining that has lost its ability to act properly as a filter. Whereas a healthy intestine allows only nutrients to pass into the bloodstream, a damaged or "leaky" one lets incompletely digested foods and bacteria get through. These substances can then provoke an immune response in other tissues and organs throughout the body. Your system may become hypersensitive to foods, and you can develop multiple food and/or environmental allergies and altered hormone activity—all of which can show up as a multitude of seemingly unrelated symptoms through your body. Vaginal, bladder, and sinus infections may be frequent. The infestation can encourage alcohol, sugar, and carbohydrate cravings. The toxins from candida affect our nervous system and can be responsible for depression, mental confusion, and even memory loss.

As candida produces more candida, your gut begins a fermentation process and an excessive amount of gas forms. Many clients say that when they eat sugar and bread—both of which contribute to candida growth—their bellies rise like bread dough and they appear four to five months pregnant (men included!). With this fermentation process, there is often diarrhea or a combination of diarrhea and constipation that is often diagnosed as irritable bowel syndrome.

Gut's Wisdom (Symptoms)

- Bloat/gas.
- Abdominal pain.
- Chronic constipation or diarrhea (irritable bowel syndrome symptoms).
- Skin problems (acne, psoriasis, eczema).
- Persistent vaginal or bladder infections.
- Athlete's foot, hair and nail fungus, jock itch.
- Multiple allergies.
- Muscular aches and/or aching joints.
- Depression and mood swings.
- Feeling "off" on damp, muggy days.
- Sensitivity to moldy places.
- Fatigue.
- PMS.
- Fuzzy and cloudy thinking.
- Sugar, bread, and alcohol cravings.
- Canker sores.
- Ear infection (congested or runny ears).
- Recurring colds and flu.
- Low libido.

This list can go on and on. Dr. Crook's book, *The Yeast Connection*, and *The Missing Diagnosis* by C. Orion Truss are suggested for a more comprehensive investigation of candida and its body-wide effects.

Contributor to Gut Dysfunction: The Gut-Brain Connection

Candida suggests a "hostile takeover" and spills old and new toxins throughout the entire body. Candida takes advantage of your gut's imbalanced state in a way that may mirror the way you relate to others or vice versa. How are your personal boundaries? Do you respect other people's boundaries? Do you speak up when others have invaded yours? Have you allowed old memories, attitudes, and emotions to remain in charge, clouding your present life's situation? Have you allowed other people to dictate how you will live? Do you feel vulnerable and unprotected? Candida overgrowth can express an inner desire to "armor" (bloat) your gut against these uncomfortable irritations.

Gut-Brain Attitudes

- Allowing the past to rule today.
- Feeling vulnerable and unprotected.
- Feeling disempowered.
- Ignoring your own needs.

Other Contributors to Gut Dysfunction

▶ **Repeated antibiotic use** is the most common cause of yeast overgrowth. Antibiotics destroy protective, friendly bacteria, leaving the gut vulnerable to candida overgrowth.

▶ **Cortisone drugs** as well as other medications may reduce the gut's defenses against yeast.

▶ **Birth control pills** stimulate yeast growth.

▶ **Poor dietary choices** can compromise your immune system. Processed foods, fast foods, excessive carbohydrates, sugars, and alcohol are a tasty smorgasbord for candida.

▶ **Alcoholism and/or eating disorders** stress the immune system as well as leave the gut's protective bacterial balance in disarray. This dysbosis (imbalanced bacteria) is a perfect breeding ground for candida.

▶ **Chronic constipation and/or diarrhea** compromise the gut's bacterial flora balance, leaving you susceptible to candida overgrowth.

▶ **Stress.** Our gut reacts to emotional, mental, and physical stress by producing less S(IgA), which is an antibody that lines our gut and protects our immune system and keeps bacteria, viruses, and yeasts at bay. Lower levels of S(IgA) mean a compromised immune system and a more vulnerable, less protected gut.

Befriending Invitations for Creating a Functional Gut

▶ **Kill the candidiasis** by not feeding the candida their favorite goodies. In order to starve those tenacious yeasts from the foods they thrive on, eliminate packaged, processed, and refined foods, all sugars, dairy, all alcohol, all foods containing yeast and vinegars, and fruit juices. Avoid all food containing molds, such as leftovers, cheese, products that contain peanuts, and mushrooms. The common therapeutic diet, which often feels quite limited, includes eggs, chicken, fish, beef, vegetable oil, nuts, and seeds. This may seem strict but remember that such a diet is only for a temporary period (three to six months)—relatively short compared to the period of time you have already suffered!

You may feel worse before feeling better due to the candida fungus dying off. "Die-off" effects are usually experienced the first two weeks of the program, with flu-like symptoms (stuffy head, headaches, general body aches, and diarrhea), skin rashes, vaginal irritation/discharge, an exacerbation of mental fog and mood swings. Colon therapy can substantially alleviate many of these symptoms. Most people feel noticeably better in about three to four weeks (if they are adhering to the protocol strictly). Candida is a tenacious critter, so it is important to stay on the program for three to six months; *listen to your gut.* You may choose to bring in other foods sooner than that. As you introduce a food you had cut out, *listen,* because your gut will speak back to you with some familiar (voices) symptoms if your candida is not in control.

▶ **Meats and poultry** should be baked or broiled. Use free-range, steroid- and antibiotic-free meats as much as possible.

▶ **Greens** are powerful immune system builders that rebalance the pH level of your intestinal tract so that candida doesn't have a place to call home. Eat plenty of green leafy vegetables (spinach, kale, collard greens), fresh green vegetable juices (use carrots or beets sparingly as they are high in sugar). Super Green tablets include chlorophyll, spirulina, alfalfa, wheat grass, and barley grass; taking them is an easy way to supplement the missing greens in your diet, as well as balance the gut's pH level. Use three to six capsules daily (combinations of all greens are available; see Appendix C).

▶ **Experiment with Wisdom Food Combining.** If you suffer from candida, your digestion is generally not working 100 percent. Correct food combining will support easier digestion, thus preventing gut fermentation, which is characterized by gas, bloating, constipation, diarrhea, and fatigue.

▸ **A Comprehensive Digestive Stool Analysis (CDSA)** is a way to check the severity of your candida (and the possibility of any other microbial factors) and guide your practitioner to what herbal or drug approach would most benefit you.

▸ **Drug therapy** may be prescribed by your health practitioner. Dyflucan, Nystatin, and Ketaconazole are potent candida killers. These have been useful for many individuals, but some side effects from these potential killers may be a suppressed immune system, so if you choose this route be sure to follow the suggestions to build your immune system and don't feed the critters.

▸ **Herbal therapy.** Grapefruit seed extract, oregano oil capsules, and olive leaf extract inhibit growth and kill the candida. They are often used successfully in the place of prescription drugs. Combinations of these herbs can be taken individually or in combinations. Take as directed.

▸ **Pau d'Arco tea** acts as an anti-fungal and can be sipped throughout the day.

▸ **Drink plenty of purified water.** Drink one quart per 50 pounds of your body weight daily. This helps flush the dead yeasts out of your body.

▸ **Gut Wisdom Cleanse** allows your system to rest, clean out, and recharge. Gut cleansing speeds the healing time and can also alleviate candida sugar cravings.

▸ **Colonics or enemas** will help remove candida from your system. Colonics are an extremely helpful adjunct therapy that provide immediate relief from gut discomforts, "mental fog," and other candida die-off reactions. If your bowels are not in top-notch condition during this time, colonics and enemas will help you to feel less uncomfortable and help facilitate a speedier recovery.

▸ **Fiber/bulk** absorbs and holds toxins within the colon and carries them out, thus reducing the toxic overload released during the treatment as the candida dies off. Experiment with different fibers and bulk, and notice which of these move your bowels most effectively. Try ground flax seed, agar, and psyllium seed husks. Take twice daily, and always follow with 8 ounces of water.

▸ **Bentonite** is a mineralized clay with powerful absorption qualities. It helps prevent the reabsorption of toxins after candida "die-off." It is like an internal poultice, drawing out and holding toxic materials. Use 1 tablespoon per 50 pounds of body weight. Mix with your bulking fiber or mix separately in water twice daily.

▸ **Brush off the past** before using steam, the sauna, or bath. Dry brushing your body all over stimulates circulation and opens skin pores to enhance toxin removal.

▸ **Sweat your toxins away.** Candida increases the toxicity of your entire body. Sweating allows your largest eliminative organ, your skin, to "move it on out." Use saunas, steam, and Epsom salts baths to facilitate your sweating and release process, complete with a *hot and cold flush.*

▸ **Acidophilus and bifidus** are necessary to reestablish normal flora in the digestive tract, leaving no room for candida to flourish. They also assist in boosting the immune system. Your elimination should improve and your ability to absorb nutrients will be enhanced. Select a highly potent, refrigerated supplement to help balance gut flora and fight the candida takeover. Take two capsules twice daily or 1/4 teaspoon of each in water twice daily.

▸ **Glutamine** is a nutrient to help repair the intestinal mucous lining (leaky gut) that is often damaged by the toxins produced by candida. Take daily for three months. Other supportive nutrients and herbs that assist in repairing the intestinal lining are deglycyrrhizinated licorice, aloe vera, slippery elm, and marshmallow root (combination formulas are available, see Appendix C).

▸ **Digestive enzymes.** If your foods are not digested thoroughly, bowel dybosis (toxicity) can result, assaulting your gut further. Also, if foods are not digested thoroughly, absorption is compromised, as well as your immune system. Use digestive enzyme tablets with each meal.

▸ **A yeast-free vitamin/mineral supplement** will help strengthen your immune system, which is needed to keep the "critters" at bay.

▸ **Herbal natural laxatives** keep the bowels moving regularly. Begin with one a day and increase as needed.

▸ **Castor oil packs.** The healing and detoxifying benefits of castor oil aid in building the strength of your digestive and eliminative systems. Apply a castor oil pack for one hour a day for three consecutive days.

▸ **Warmth on your belly.** Using the Belly Buddy or a hot water bottle on your belly brings blood and nutrients that aid in healing. Warmth is both emotionally protective and nurturing to a vulnerable gut area.

▸ **Belly massage** helps move out trapped gases and stool. Massage stimulates the "feel-good" healing endorphins.

▶ **Belly breathing** helps reduce stress. The body can then begin a healing and restorative process, and proper bowel function can be supported.

▶ **Exercise and wisdom-cises** oxygenate your body and assist in reducing the damaging affects of stress buildup.

▶ **Embracing and conversations with your gut** are beneficial befriending gestures to use to explore what your gut needs to restore your inner strength. This process encourages you to listen and begin building a functional relationship with your gut.

▶ **A wisdom journal** and/or support from a qualified counselor who will help you to see what past, discomforting, immune-suppressing experiences you might be bringing into the present. Are you willing to take charge of your personal boundaries and needs? Are you willing to empower yourself and be present in today's experiences? Or will the past continue to poison you?

▶ **Be gentle** and as nonjudgmental as possible as you explore and become aware of what lurks within you. Remember: With awareness comes the opportunity for change.

▶ **Thank your gut** for the guidance it has bestowed upon you to strengthen personal boundaries and stand empowered within yourself.

Diarrhea
What Is It?

Talk about something running your life: Those with diarrhea are inhibited no matter where they are by the fear of unexpected bowel discharge. Diarrhea is often your gut's way of getting rid of something that is not agreeing with it.

Diarrhea is a condition of frequent, loose, watery stools that come with an unexpected and sometimes uncontrollable urge to become one with a toilet. It may include cramping, thirst, and/or vomiting and fever. Most of us have diarrhea from time to time—maybe you ate some tainted food, indulged a bit too much with celebratory spirits, or just got a bug. However, *chronic* diarrhea is what we are talking about (although the following suggestions are for a mild case as well).

If diarrhea is chronic or ongoing, it can rob the body of water, salts, potassium, and other precious electrolytes (minerals). Due to the rapid transit of stool, your foods cannot be absorbed properly, which can lead to malnutrition—not at all good for your overall health.

Gut's Wisdom (Symptoms)

- Constant loose stool.
- Abdominal cramping.
- Thirst.
- Fever.
- Nausea.

Contributor to Gut Dysfunction: The Gut-Brain Connection

With diarrhea, the small or large intestine may be involved. The small intestine is our assimilator and separator of what is pure and impure physically, mentally, and emotionally. The large intestine is our holding tank, where we discard what no longer serves us. Are you rushing, wanting to get things over with rather than taking time to "smell the roses" and to feel nourished in this moment? Are you *running* to what's next mentally or emotionally? What or who are you attempting to "expel" or reject from your life or do you fear you are being rejected?

If cramping occurs, there is a constriction or spasm of the gut. This is a "drawing in," a possible "holding on" and fear of not being in control (which we all would like to think we are).

Gut-Brain Attitudes

- Anxiety about the "what ifs" or "should haves."
- Unable to receive (emotional) nourishment.
- Fear of losing control.
- Rejection: feeling rejected or wanting to reject.

Other Contributors to Gut Dysfunction

▶ **Food poisoning** occurs from eating contaminated food. Parasites or bacteria such as salmonella, E-coli, and campylobacter, can be found in contaminated eggs, dairy products, poultry or fish.

▶ **Lactose intolerance** can contribute to diarrhea.

▶ **Hormonal changes** prior to or during the menstrual cycle are often accompanied with a bout of diarrhea.

▶ **Foe foods** that you are sensitive or allergic to or are just not right for your gut can respond with diarrhea. Some of the main culprits are dairy, wheat and other gluten grains, fats (fried or rich foods), sugar, and alcohol.

▶ **Irritable bowel syndrome**'s voice is usually constipation followed with diarrhea. Ingesting irritable bowel syndrome foe foods (see "Irritable Bowel Syndrome on page 201) can exacerbate the condition.

▶ **Medications/drugs** often have a side effect of diarrhea. Antibiotics and antacids disrupt our gut's friendly bacteria balance, and diarrhea becomes an uncomfortable result.

▶ **Gall bladder** imbalances can contribute to diarrhea, due to the organ's inability to assist in properly digesting fats.

▶ **Candida** is a yeast/fungus that naturally resides in your gut in small amounts. When your gut is compromised by illness, antibiotics, foe foods, and stress, candida proliferates, and diarrhea is often one of a multitude of gut voices (symptoms).

▶ **Vitamins and minerals** in excess can be a diarrhea contributor. Ingesting large amounts of vitamin C and/or magnesium can make your bowels runny.

▶ **Parasites** such as Giardia cause diarrhea. It can be contracted from contaminated water, foods, daycare centers, and pets or during travel.

▶ **Stress and anxiety** activate your nervous system, as well as your bowels.

▶ **Constipation.** This boggles many people's minds, but if your stool is stuck in your colon, your gut's wisdom will do its best to attempt to draw water into the colon to give you your own personal "enema/colonic" to move the stool out.

Befriending Invitations for Creating a Functional Gut

▶ If **diarrhea** persists for longer than a week, see your doctor.

▶ **Omit foe foods.** Examine what you eat daily. Diarrhea is a common gut voice of food sensitivities and/or allergies. Omit one food completely at a time for a week. Listen to your gut; it will speak. The biggest culprits are dairy, fats, gluten grains (wheat, rye, oats, barley), sugar, alcohol, caffeine, and spicy foods. You may also choose to see your health provider for allergy blood tests.

▶ **Include friendly foods:** vegetables, legumes, fruits, plain yogurt, tofu, chicken, fish, and whole grains. Follow the Wisdom Diet.

▶ **Acidophilus and bifidus** replenish the lost friendly bacteria and help normalize bowel function. Use a nondairy form, two capsules, three times daily or 1/4 teaspoon powder twice daily.

▸ **Activated charcoal tablets** absorb the toxins from your colon. Take three to four tablets every hour until the diarrhea is alleviated. Take separately from your other medications and supplements. Don't be alarmed when your bowel movements appear black; it is only the charcoal. Alternatively, *bentonite* is a volcanic ash (it's safe for children—I was raised on this product!) that absorbs 10 times its weight in toxins. Take the recommended amount (one teaspoon per 50 pounds of body weight; taken in 8 ounces of filtered water) every two or three hours.

▸ **Digestive enzymes** help you digest and allow you to assimilate the nutrients from your food and help minimize further gut irritation and gas. Take with each meal.

▸ **Multivitamin and mineral supplements** (in the appropriate amounts) replenish lost nutrients. Use daily as directed.

▸ **Fluids** are important to ingest to prevent dehydration. Including fresh green vegetable juices and Wisdom Broth is an excellent way to replenish the loss of valuable minerals that can occur with diarrhea. Ginger tea is comforting for cramps and abdominal pain.

▸ **Bulking fibers** such as ground flax seed or psyllium or Metamucil help solidify stool. Start with 1 1/2 teaspoon in 8 ounces of water; increase to 1 tablespoon.

▸ **Warming your belly** with a Belly Buddy or hot water bottle helps calm and soothe an overactive bowel and is comforting for a cramping ailing belly.

▸ **Belly breathing** calms an agitated nervous system and allows restoration and healing to take place.

▸ **Belly massage** is calming and soothing to an overworked gut. It can assist in relaxing the "gripping" in the gut as a result of bowel muscles being in spasm.

▸ **Gut Wisdom Cleanse** can clean out "internal irritants" and can restore gut balance in a short period of time.

▸ If the diarrhea is chronic, ask your health practitioner for a **Comprehensive Digestive Stool Test (CDSA)** to check for digestive and eliminative imbalances, parasites, or candida.

▸ **Embracing and conversation with the gut** can compassionately guide you to what held emotions and attitudes may be contributing to the diarrhea.

▶ **Slow down.** Take time in your life to fully experience whatever is occurring so you can "absorb" and obtain the full benefits and blessing of the present moment.

▶ **Assist in the process of letting go and forgiving.** Let go of the beliefs and attitudes around control.

▶ A **forgiveness ceremony** could be a beneficial step in your healing process. Be open to receive. Take in the love and nourishment that surround you.

▶ **Thank your gut** for speaking up and offering an indication that there is a need for some physical or emotional new choices.

Diverticulosis

What Is It?

Give any muscle enough pressure and it begins to distort. Just like a bubble blown from a piece of chewing gum, gas and waste (fecal matter) can blow out weakened intestinal walls in pea-sized pouches called diverticula. The underlying contributor of diverticula formation is constipation. Compacted, hard, dehydrated waste is difficult for intestines to move along. Chronic constipation can put an increased pressure on the intestinal walls, resulting in diverticular pouches. Diverticulosis can occur along the small or large intestine but are most often found in the descending and sigmoid portion of the colon (left side).

In the 1950s, diverticulosis only affected 10 percent of U.S. adults older than 45. In 1987, almost 50 percent of the U.S. population was diagnosed with this condition. According to the *Merck Manual,* the most recent report predicts that *everyone* will be diagnosed with diverticulosis at some point after the age of 40 (are they betting our diets won't change?).

One can have diverticulosis and be basically symptom-free with the exception of some mild gas and bloating. However, problems occur when waste becomes stuck and stagnant in the diverticuli. As bacteria proliferates and inflammation occurs, the condition changes to a condition called diverticulitis. The toxins that accompany the inflamed pouches may absorb into our system and result in autointoxication (self-poisoning).

With a diverticulitis attack*, gas, fever, and abdominal pain occur due to the irritation and inflammation of the bowel membrane.* Sometimes these inflamed pouches may heal on their own, especially with the implementation of dietary changes, supplements, and gut-brain befriending techniques. Unfortunately, if the condition is serious, antibiotics may be necessary. If there is a ruptured diverticula, surgery may be the only option.

Gut's Wisdom (Symptoms)

- Gas.
- Constipation and/or alternating diarrhea.
- Cramping.
- Distended abdominal area.
- Nausea.

Diverticulitis (if diverticuli are inflamed) you could experience all of these symptoms plus:

- Chills.
- Fevers.
- Abdominal pain.
- Blood in stool.
- Tenderness on left side of abdomen.
- Irritable bowel syndrome symptoms.

Contributors to Gut Dysfunction: The Gut-Brain Connection

Diverticulosis affects our large intestine, which is our "holding tank," a place for our waste to hang out for a moment as all of "what no longer serves us" passes through and, hopefully, out. With diverticulosis, our leftovers, so to speak, get trapped. Our stagnant waste-filled diverticuli reflect holding on to old ideas, self-limiting beliefs, attitudes, and emotions that should be over and done with.

When the waste gets trapped and stagnate in the diverticuli, it begins to putrefy, causing gas, bloat, constipation, and irritation. Stagnation in the bowel often reflects a refusal or fear of letting go. Trust comes into the picture here: "If I let go, then what? Will I be safe?" You may unconsciously feel you need that tenderness and bloat to armor and protect those old vulnerable (now toxic) feelings.

Often cramping accompanies diverticulosis, which may signify emotional holding on, drawing up, and mistrusting. When the condition has reached the diverticulitis (inflammation) stage, your gut is screaming to get your attention and possibly informing you that *letting go* is an important step on your healing journey.

Gut-Brain Attitudes

- Feeling "trapped" in areas of your life.
- Harboring aggravations toward others or self.
- Difficulty in letting go of past emotional grievances.
- Difficulty in letting go of unhealthy attitudes and beliefs.

Other Contributors to Gut Dysfunction

▶ **Constipation** is a major contributor to diverticular disease. This usually accompanies a diet lacking in sufficient fiber and water. Without fiber and water, our stools are harder to pass, increasing pressure on the intestinal wall and causing diverticular pouches.

▶ **Foe foods** such as refined flour products (pastries, breads, pasta, cakes) are low on the fiber totem pole, high on the mucous scale, and high in sugar that feeds unfriendly bacteria. These foods can exacerbate constipation and inflammation.

▶ **Any chronic disease** that weakens the smooth muscle can leave the bowel muscles weakened and susceptible to pouch formation.

Befriending Invitations for Creating a Functional Gut

▶ **Avoid foe foods** such as fried foods, sugars, dairy, low-fiber foods, red meat, and spicy foods so as not to continue to weaken and constipate the bowel.

▶ **Avoid nuts and seed foods,** such as sesame seeds, cucumbers, strawberries. The seeds and nuts may get caught and irritate in your diverticuli.

▶ **Include friendly fiber foods** by increasing your intake of vegetables, fruits, legumes, and non-gluten whole grains (brown rice, quinoa, amaranth). Follow the Gut Wisdom Diet.

▶ **Supplement with fiber products** such as ground flax seed, psyllium husk powder, or Metamucil twice daily to get/keep stools bulky, soft, and gentle to pass. Increasing water is also a must when using bulking products.

▶ **Get juiced.** Fresh green vegetable juices are rich in chlorophyll and very soothing and healing for the gut's lining. A supportive combination is spinach, kale, and broccoli, sweetened with a little carrot and/or a slice of apple. Use 2 tablespoons of liquid chlorophyll per 8 ounces of water if vegetable juices are unavailable.

▶ **Acidophilus and bifidus** are friendly gut protectors that can help fight infection, inflammation, and gas that may occur as waste gets stuck in the diverticuli. Use a nondairy form, two capsules, three times daily or 1/4 teaspoon powder twice daily.

▶ **Aloe vera juice** is a digestive system healer. It has anti-inflammatory properties, is extremely soothing to the intestinal lining, and will help relieve constipation. Drink 1/2 cup daily on an empty stomach daily.

▶ **Pau d'Arco tea** is an antibacterial cleansing tea that helps inhibit bacterial overgrowth and inflammation. Drink 2 to 3 cups daily.

▶ **Take a comprehensive enzyme** to help support digestion of your foods that will in turn prevent further gut irritation and enhance elimination. Include one capsule with each meal.

▶ **L-Glutamine, deglycyrrhizinated licorice, slippery elm, and marshmallow root** assist in the repair and restoration of the mucosal intestinal lining. Recommended usage of this combination is 1/2 teaspoon three times daily for three months and is available from your professional health practitioner (Intestinal Repair Complex, see Appendix C).

▶ **Castor oil packs** applied to the tender area can help reduce inflammation. Apply over the abdomen (with extra focus on the left side) for one hour a day, three days in a row. This can help loosen stuck waste matter and has been reported to significantly reduce the inflammation.

▶ Use **belly breathing** can help relieve associated discomforts.

▶ **Belly massage** with extra attention on the left side of the abdomen. Remember to breathe deeply as you massage. Apply a hot water bottle or Belly Buddy to bring soothing comfort and help restore blood and healing nutrients to the affected area.

▶ **Wisdom squat** to stimulate and encourage an easy bowel movement.

▶ **Colon therapy** helps clear out the waste, excessive gases, and toxins, thus preventing further pressure in the diverticula.

▶ **Gut Wisdom Cleanse** can clean out the stuck and stagnant waste and gases, preventing further gut damage from occurring. It's an opportunity to become increasingly aware of the effects that your food choices have on your gut's health.

▶ **Hot/cold flush** each morning on your abdomen can bring fresh blood and stimulation to the present stagnant areas in your gut.

▶ **Movement** begets movement. Exercise and gut releasing stretches unstick us!

▶ **Let go of the old.** Are you feeling stuck in a dead-end job or relationship? Are you willing to move forward? Who or what aggravates you? Where are you feeling trapped in your life? Which situations, experiences, or feelings are you *holding on* to?

▶ **Forgiveness ceremony.** Who needs forgiving and letting go? You? Them? The forgiveness ceremony may be in order to help you in this process of letting go.

▶ **Using embracing and conversations with the gut** can both comfort and awaken you to what your gut message is and how to attend to it physically and emotionally.

▶ **Wisdom journal** can help you move out all those toxic feelings, attitudes, beliefs in a safe way.

▶ **Thank your gut wisdom** for its voice of guidance and its desire to direct you towards health.

Befriending Invitations for a Diverticulitis Attack

▶ **See your doctor.** An antibiotic may be prescribed or some diagnostic testing may be required (a barium enema with an X-ray or a sigmoidoscopy).

▶ You may safely take **acidophilus and bifidus** to reduce some of the inflammation. If you are taking antibiotics, see "How to Replenish Friendly Bacteria During Your Antibiotic Treatment" in Chapter 7.

▶ With a diverticulitis attack, **low fiber** is recommended until the attack is over. Puree your foods, and steam and bake vegetables. Broth or health food store baby foods are other options.

▶ **Activated charcoal** can be taken to absorb excessive and painful gas. Try two to three capsules three times daily.

▶ **A castor oil pack** is a magic healer and soother of gut inflammation. Use it for one to one and a half hours, three days in a row.

▶ **Aloe vera juice** can help soothe the irritated intestinal lining. Use 1/2 cup per day.

▶ **L-Glutamine, deglycyrrhized licorice, slippery elm, and marshmallow root** provide nutrients to repair and soothe the intestinal lining. Recommended usage of this combination is 1/2 teaspoon three times daily for three months and is available from your professional health practitioner (Intestinal Repair Complex, see Appendix C).

▶ **Avoid laxatives;** they will only aggravate your condition.

▶ **Check for any food allergies** that may contribute to gut irritations and inflammations.

▶ **Letting go,** forgiving, embracing, journaling, and getting support are highlighted in diverticulitis, because your gut's wisdom is basically screaming at you to pay attention.

Hemorrhoids

What Are They?

More than 75 percent of Americans will experience hemorrhoids at some point in their lives. By the age of 50, as many as half of the U.S. population has experienced this condition. Hemorrhoid treatment is a $50-million-a-year industry. Preparation H, which is used to reduce hemorrhoidal inflammation, is the fourth most popular over-the-counter remedy. We are the only creatures that develop this anal challenge. Might this be saying something about our diets and lifestyles?

Hemorrhoids are swollen veins that can occur internally or externally in the anus and rectum. *Internal hemorrhoids* are located inside your rectum. Usually one doesn't know he or she has them unless the hemorrhoids break or rupture with bright-colored blood appearing on the toilet paper, in the toilet, or mixed in with the stool.

External hemorrhoids protrude outside the anal sphincter. These often become engorged with blood, making it painful to sit or have a bowel movement. Other symptoms include burning, itching, inflammation, swelling, seepage and sometimes bleeding and downright pain!

Remember: You're not alone. Napoleon is said to have suffered from hemorrhoids on the battlefield—and he had to ride a horse. Ouch!

Gut's Wisdom (Symptoms)

- Rectal pain.
- Rectal itching.
- Rectal bleeding with bowel movement.
- Swollen protrusions in or around the anus.

Contributors to Gut Dysfunction: The Gut-Brain Connection

Hemorrhoids are located at our final porthole. We accumulate waste that has served its purpose and needs to be let out for the sake of our gut, body, and mind. It is an act of surrendering and letting go.

Hemorrhoid pain, discomfort, and/or irritation may be reflecting a difficulty you have in letting go of a situation or feeling that needs to be released. Your hemorrhoid may be a painful reminder to you and inviting you to let go. *If there is persistent bleeding, see a doctor. Persistent bleeding can lead to anemia or indicate other serious problems. Do not ignore bleeding!*

Gut-Brain Attitudes

- Difficulty letting go of past attitudes, beliefs, or experiences.
- Irritated by an individual or situation.
- Unfulfilled desire (itch) in your life.

Other Contributors to Gut Dysfunction

▸ **Repeated straining** as one attempts to have a bowel movement creates pressure and forces blood to engorge into the hemorrhoidal vein.

▸ A **low-fiber diet, inadequate water, and foe foods** can contribute to constipation that can result in hemorrhoids forming.

▸ **Lack of exercise** is frequently accompanied by lack of proper bowel functioning.

▸ **Prolonged periods of sitting, standing, and/or lifting heavy objects.**

▸ **Pregnancy and childbirth.** Just about every mom will speak of her hemorrhoids due to the additional pressure on the abdomen and anus, compounded by the delivery of "Junior" as well as the constipation that often accompanies pregnancy.

Befriending Invitations for Creating a Functional Gut

▸ Go directly to "Constipation" on page 172 and attend to the primary problem.

▸ Dietary revisions are suggested. **Increase your intake of fiber** and bulk, whole grains, fruits, vegetables, legumes, ground flax seed, oat bran, psyllium, or Metamucil, and increase your water consumption daily. Omit foe foods and substances. Follow the Gut Wisdom Diet and include gut-befriending supplements (acidophilus, bifidus, and digestive enzymes).

▸ **Wisdom squat** to eliminate further straining on your rectal muscles.

▸ Take **vitamin E suppositories** (Carlson Labs) for pain and itching. Taking a vitamin E supplement orally will help bring oxygen to the affected rectal tissues to support healing.

▸ Apply **salves, ointment, or oil** to a cotton ball and apply to the hemorrhoids to reduce inflammation. Suggested: castor oil, vitamin E oil, calendula ointment, goldenseal, or comfrey salves.

▸ Use a **kinder, softer toilet paper** to prevent any further irritation.

▸ **Vitamin C complex** with bioflavanoids and rutin strengthen blood vessels and capillaries to assist in further rupturing. Vitamin C will also soften the stools and encourage a gentler bowel movement. Recommended dosage is 1,000–2,000 milligrams daily.

▸ **Movement** (exercise, wisdom-cises) helps encourage bowel regularity.

▸ **Belly breathing** assists in keeping your bowels functioning efficiently.

▶ **The Gut Wisdom Cleanse** will give your gut and hemorrhoids a chance to heal.

▶ **Express your thoughts and feelings** and then let go, so as not to "hold on."

▶ **Forgiveness ceremony and journaling** are each supportive, befriending tools to assist in letting go.

▶ **Change your attitude** to one of acceptance and forgiveness. Get the person or situation that is a "pain in your butt" out of your life, or alter your attitude toward that person or situation.

▶ **Embracing and conversation with gut** can help you compassionately understand and heal what is the message and what your gut (and butt) needs for relief.

▶ **Thank your hemorrhoids** for the nudge of guidance they are offering you to let go.

Indigestion

What Is It?

Burp, gas, bloat, heartburn—they are all cries for relief. Good gut health is difficult to achieve without good digestion. Heartburn, gastric reflux, gas, bloat and belching are messages that our digestive process is not working properly.

When the gut is malfunctioning, nutrients aren't sufficiently absorbed, which makes you susceptible to other health challenges. Poor digestion contributes to food sensitivities, allergies, and gut challenges further down the line (constipation, IBS, lower bowel gas, fatigue, and more).

Heartburn

Heartburn is experienced as a burning sensation above the stomach and/or chest and sometimes is mistaken for a heart attack. One third of Americans experience heartburn, and the number of sufferers has been increasing steadily. Hmm...could it be our lifestyles?

Of course, the first thing that most of us do when this burning occurs is to listen to the media's modern medicine solution: pop the antacid. This approach may quiet the gut's persistent voices, temporarily, but antacids often mask an underlying problem.

Heartburn is caused by stomach acid backing up into your esophagus, accompanied with burning sensations, regurgitation, belching, and a sour taste in the mouth.

When diets are shifted to healthier, high-fiber choices, the heartburn will often dissipate—a message from your gut that perhaps the trouble is not too much stomach acid but too many foe foods. Smoking and excess weight can also exacerbate symptoms.

The food in your stomach needs to be digested thoroughly and properly. For your stomach to do its job, it needs hydrochloric acid (HCl). Believe it or not, your heartburn is generally *not* caused by too much acid. A lack of HCl in your stomach causes a fermentation and bloat to occur. The sensation that follows feels like a burning eruption, with a few belches and a possible sour taste in your mouth. The pressure of gases in your stomach pushes the valve at the end of your esophagus, and some of your dinner's contents are allowed to wash up into your esophagus. Antacids will offer only temporary relief. The stomach's natural reaction to this acid repression is to balance itself by making more acid. This is called *acid rebound*. If the antacids are overused, eventually very little acid is made. But you leave yourself depleted of natural HCl and other digestive complications may follow:

> ⊳ **Inability to digest protein,** which leads to malabsorption of other nutrients, more gas, bloat, heartburn, and allergies. (Most allergies are the result of incompletely digested proteins that enter the bloodstream and cause an antibody reaction.)

> ⊳ **Inability of the stomach acid** to kill unfriendly bacteria like it should. This can lead to "unfriendly" microorganisms affecting your gut's health.

> ⊳ **Stomach acids** help you absorb calcium, and iron. Lack of these nutrients can contribute to osteoporosis and anemia, respectively.

Gastric Reflux

Normally, the esophageal sphincter muscle pinches itself shut to prevent our stomach acid from surging upward and visiting you. However, if the sphincter is not functioning according to our gut design, *gastric reflux* (gastroesophageal reflux) occurs, which is when the acid sneaks past the sphincter into the esophagus, causing a burning and scarring of the tissues as well as problems swallowing.

Hiatal Hernia

This is a condition in which part of the stomach is pushed upward (herniates) through the diaphragm into the chest cavity. The symptoms of hiatal hernia include heartburn, belching, and gastroesophogeal reflux (gastric reflux). A person suffering a hiatal hernia may experience difficulty in swallowing. With all these symptoms, the tissues in the esophagus become irritated. If symptoms are persistent, a scarring as well as ulceration of the esophagus and stomach may occur.

Gas, Bloating, and Belching

Gas is a normal fact of life. When excessive, however, it causes discomfort and distention of the abdominal area. Excessive gas bloating and belching are often signs that our food is not digesting sufficiently and fermentation and/or putrefaction is present.

Gut's Wisdom (Symptoms)

- Burning sensation in or above the stomach after eating.

- Sour or bitter taste in the mouth.

- Belching.

- Excess gas.

- Fullness in the stomach for a prolonged period of time.

- Bloat.

- A pain in the chest area.

- Difficulty swallowing.

Contributor to Dysfunction: The Gut-Brain Connection

Heartburn, gastric reflux, hiatal hernia, and gas can stem from an imbalance in the stomach. Taoist sages called the stomach the "sea of nourishment." It represents a place to "take in." We take in new thoughts, ideas, experiences, and feelings in order to digest, process, break down, and assimilate them into our beings and our life. We depend on a reliable constant source of physical, emotional, and spiritual nourishment to be balanced and healthy individuals.

Our guts' voice (symptoms) may speak if we encounter a situation that may be "hard to swallow," "hard to stomach," or "unpalatable" to fully "digest" (process, understand, accept, or believe). This stress can cause our nervous system to react in fight-or-flight response, hindering our digestive and elimination function.

A hiatal hernia is a "rupture" in the diaphragm (over our solar plexus, our seat of emotion). What unexpressed feelings need to be expressed? Anger and frustration may be repressed as you and your diaphragm attempt to hold down tight and keep control of those feelings. The wisdom of your gut might keep pushing up to remind you to honor, feel, and express your feelings and then let go!

Who or what situation/person is irritating or "burning you up?" Have you expressed it? Are there situations/feelings that are difficult for you to "digest" and often seem to regurgitate back by repetitive, obsessive thoughts? Are you able to allow others to nourish you, to receive love and care without resistance? Do you have a difficult time taking in ideas and concepts and then putting them into action? What's "hard to swallow?"

Gut-Brain Attitudes

- Anxiety or fear.
- Difficulty in expressing anger and/or frustration.
- A situation, person, or memory is "burning" at you.
- Unable to "stomach" an experience, idea, or information you've received.

Other Contributors to Gut Dysfunction

▸ **Eating when stressed** inhibits proper digestion that causes gas in the intestines or in the stomach. The gas may push up against your esophageal sphincter, giving an opportunity for stomach acids to flush upward.

▸ **Poor food combinations.** Research has shown that starches (breads, potatoes, sugar) and proteins (meat, fish, eggs, and poultry) require different enzymes for digestion. Combining these foods in a single meal can slow down your digestion, causing gas, bloating, and heartburn.

▸ **Foe foods** or, better said, tasty-but-not-necessarily-good-for-you-and-your-gut foods. Fried or fatty food, alcohol, coffee, spicy, and/or refined foods (junk) can irritate your stomach. If your stomach is already irritated, citrus fruits, tomato-based foods, sodas, and sugars can add to the irritation.

▸ **Overeating** taxes your digestive and eliminative system. If you "can't believe you ate the whole thing," you ate too much and your system cannot digest the overload.

▸ **Food allergies,** parasites, candida, constipation, and disorders of the pancreas, liver, or gallbladder can all contribute to a variety of indigestion symptoms.

▸ **Low stomach acid.** Hydrochloric acid (HCl) is a common cause of indigestion. Most individuals older than 50 have low HCl levels in their stomachs. Symptoms include belching, bloat, and a feeling that food has overstayed its welcome in your stomach.

▶ **Lactose intolerance** is a malabsorption condition, caused by a deficiency of the enzyme lactase. Lactose intolerance can be the culprit in bloating and abdominal gas (see the "Lactose Intolerance" section in this chapter).

▶ **Medications** such as antibiotics, Nicotine, Diazepam, and Provera can contribute to heartburn.

▶ **Helicobacter pylori (H-pylori)** is a bacteria that has been associated in gastric ulcer and has been implicated in many cases of gastric reflux. See your doctor for an evaluation.

▶ **Constipation/straining** to have a bowel movement can herniate the stomach through the diaphragm. Dr. Neal Barnard, author of *The Power of Your Plate,* states: "We have never found any community in the world which passes large, soft stools and gets hiatal hernias."

Befriending Invitations for Creating a Functional Gut

▶ **Digestive support** for stomach gas, belching, a bloated feeling, and a burning sensation after eating (excluding if you have an ulcer) may be relieved by supplementing your diet with a digestive enzyme tablet that includes hydrochloric acid (HCl). Insufficient amounts of HCl can contribute to indigestion. To determine whether you need more HCl, take a tablespoon of apple cider vinegar in a glass of water. If this dissipates your indigestion, this is a sign that your stomach is not creating HCl. If it makes your symptoms worse, then you have too much acid and should avoid digestive enzymes.

▶ **Omit foe, irritating foods** such as fried, processed, or spicy foods, red meat, alcohol, coffee, sugars, or carbonated beverages.

▶ **Check with your doctor** to confirm that the medication you are taking is not contributing to your discomfort.

▶ **Keep a careful Wisdom Food Journal.** Omit at least one foe food culprit at a time for three to 10 days and notice how your gut feels. You may choose to reintroduce the suspected culprit into your diet. Listen to your gut. It will voice its opinion if this is one of the culprits.

▶ **Follow the Gut Wisdom Diet** program.

▶ **Eat small amounts of food** more frequently throughout the day.

▶ **Chew your foods completely** to help prevent excessive gas.

▶ **Limit or omit fluids with your meals.** This dilutes the stomach enzyme and prevents good digestion.

▶ **At the first signs of heartburn**, drink 8 ounces of water to dilute excess acid.

▶ **Use activated charcoal capsules** for occasional relief. Charcoal is great for absorbing gas and toxins but may also interfere with absorption of valuable nutrients and medications, so use it sparingly.

▶ **Use aloe vera juice** to soothe an inflamed stomach or esophagus. Recommendation: Drink 1/2 cup daily until symptoms subside.

▶ **Drink soothing herbal teas** such as slippery elm, Pau d'Arco, or marshmallow to soothe inflamed stomach tissues.

▶ **Omit smoking,** which can contribute to your gut irritation.

▶ **Omit aspirin,** which can contribute to your gut irritation.

▶ **Chiropractic and osteopathic treatment** can restore diaphragm muscle tone. In people with hiatal hernia, strengthening the diaphragm can help prevent acid reflux and heartburn.

▶ A **Wisdom Cleanse** may be in order (see Chapter 9) to detox your system and get back on track. It's a "must do" when you are ready to help your gut to the next level of health. The cleanse will deepen your awareness of the cause and effect of your food choices.

▶ **Colonics** are a very quick way to remove the unwanted gas and bloat. Come in with a bloated and gassy belly and leave without it.

▶ **Use daily acidophilus and bifidus.** The more that this protective friendly bacteria inhabits your gut, the less gas and stomach irritation you will experience.

▶ **Belly Breathing** is beneficial in keeping you relaxed as you eat and digest. Deep breathing is a great stress-reducer. The less stress, the better the digestion.

▶ **Apply warmth to the abdomen** to bring blood back to the digestive system, supporting the function of your digestion. Use the Belly Buddy or a hot water bottle during and after eating.

▶ **If you are experiencing constipation,** attend to this problem (see the "Constipation" section on page 172). The cleaner the colon is, the less opportunity for gas and bloat to push up and out of you.

▶ **Embracing and conversations with the gut** can help give you valuable insight as to what is "burning" to emerge.

▶ **Be aware and explore** the emotional component of what/who is "unpalatable." Take an honest look at how easy or how difficult it is to "take in" new thoughts, ideas, and attitudes and then to utilize and implement them. Reflect on how well you are nourishing yourself physically, emotionally, and spiritually.

▶ **Thank your gut** for its wisdom and its burning desire to "speak" to you.

Irritable Bowel Syndrome (IBS)

What Is It?

"Oh, my aching gut" is what millions of Americans say. Irritable bowel syndrome has become the most common digestive disorder seen by physicians. It is estimated that approximately one in five adults have symptoms of IBS, and twice as many women's gut's wisdom speak up with this condition. IBS is also sometimes called spastic colon, colitis, or ulcerative colitis.

IBS may manifest as difficult or infrequent bowel movements (constipation) and an urge to move the bowels with little success or no success at all. Others have frequent and urgent loose bowel movements. Some people alternate between diarrhea and constipation. These symptoms are often accompanied with abdominal cramps, bloat, nausea, and sometimes painful, trapped gas. Because of the unpredictability or severity of the gut's wisdom (symptoms), it has kept many people from social events, business engagements, and traveling. Some people even become hesitant to eat for fear of experiencing symptoms. Needless to say, anxiety and depression are often associated with this gut condition.

In some cases, intestinal membranes become irritated, tender, and often inflamed. In the case of colitis, mucus may be found in the stool. Ulcerative colitis is often accompanied by blood mixed with mucous because the ulcerations that line the sides of the intestine have been irritated. Symptoms may be triggered by stress or caused by eating foe foods.

Gut's Wisdom (Symptoms)

- Abdominal pain, tenderness, cramping, and spasms.
- Constipation alternating with diarrhea.
- Thin, ribbon-like or small, pebble-like bowel movements.
- Sensation of incomplete bowel movement.
- Trapped gas.
- Mucus in your stool.
- Intolerance of certain foods.
- Bloated, distended abdomen.
- Nausea.
- Anxiety.
- Depression.

Contributors to Gut Dysfunction: The Gut-Brain Connection

As stated previously, our brain can upset the gut and visa versa. As Taoist sages state, we hold and digest not just food but also our emotions in our gut. This isn't called irritable bowel syndrome by chance! If you are experiencing or holding on to irritations, angers, grief, sadness, or fears, the gut responds in kind. It is associated with maintaining power and our personal boundaries or with letting go and surrendering control.

Who or what is irritating you? What past/present anger, grief, injustices are still stirring in you? Are you feeling out of control or fearful? Do you feel safe to freely express your feelings, or do you feel you need to protect and armor your gut's vulnerable emotional center? What are you holding on to so dearly that it is getting distorted and twisted?

Gut-Brain Attitudes

- Irritated, angry, or frustrated.
- Feeling trapped.
- Lacking trust to surrender to life's experiences.
- Difficulty or fear of letting go.
- Internalized tension.
- Desire to protect vulnerable feelings.
- Rejection (rejecting others or fear of being rejected).

Other Contributors to Gut Dysfunction

▶ **Stress is a major contributor:** Many conventional doctors and internists have yet to diagnose an organic cause (virus, bacteria) but many agree that a majority of IBS can be accelerated by emotional, stress-related causes. IBS sufferers may have a gut more sensitive to stresses, possibly due to abnormalities in the nervous system. As you have learned, emotions lead to biochemical and hormonal reactions in our gut and body, which can contribute or exacerbate our gut's distress. As your nervous system flips into "stress response," your gut shuts down (constipation) or acts up (diarrhea), your digestion is altered, and abdominal tension and cramping are voiced.

▶ **Gut troublemakers,** such as antibiotics, laxatives, antacids, and medications, alter the gut's friendly bacterial flora can contribute and exacerbate gut ailments.

▶ **Foe foods** that cause sensitivities or allergies can trigger IBS.

▶ **Overindulging and not having sufficient digestive enzymes** to assist in the digestion process can cause cramping, bloating, gas, diarrhea, and gut irritation.

▶ **Hormones** may increase symptoms. Research has found that women with IBS may have more flare-ups during their menstrual periods.

▶ **Creepy crawlers** such as parasites and candida can dominate our innards and can mimic each and every symptom of IBS. Dr. Leo Galland, author of *Four Pillars of Health,* has found that the parasite Giardia was responsible for approximately half of his patients' suffering from IBS.

▶ **Lack of exercise** can allow stress to build up. Our digestive and eliminative functions suffer from the couch-potato syndrome.

Befriending Inuitations for Creating a Functional Gut

▶ **Omit foe foods,** particularly wheat (breads and pasta), gluten, dairy (due to lactose intolerance), and alcohol. Also omit coffee, sugar, and fried and high-fat foods. I've seen some of the greatest changes in clients' guts when they omit these foods. Sorry—I know these are "staples" in many people's diets. Many of you would give me your first born before letting go of your wine or that pasta dish. When you are ready, just experiment one food at a time for at least one week. If you bring that foe food back into your diet, let your gut decide.

▶ **Friendly foods** from the Gut Wisdom Diet are suggested. Veggies are important, but sometimes raw vegetables may be hard for someone with IBS to digest. Choose steamed, baked, grilled, or stir-fried veggies instead of salads.

▶ **Fiber.** Incorporate a gentle "bulking" fiber to soothe the lining of your gut and "kindly" move waste out. Choose one of the following.

　▷ **Ground flax seed.** Begin with 1 tablespoon, increase to 3 tablespoons mixed with cereal (gluten-free) or fruit or vegetable juices or sprinkled over vegetables.

　▷ **Metamucil.** (Follow as directed.)

　▷ **Psyllium husks**. (If you are chronically constipated, this should not be used.)

▶ **Wisdom Food Combining** assists in proper digestion, which helps with easier elimination.

▶ **Increase water intake** daily to eight glasses to ensure your bowels are sufficiently hydrated, thus preventing constipation.

▶ **Use acidophilus and bifidus** to replenish friendly intestinal bacteria. These help reduce gas and inflammation as well as encourage proper bowel function.

▸ **Use multivitamin and mineral capsules** to help strengthen your immune system.

▸ **Omega-3 and omega-6 oils** are essential fatty acids that inhibit the formation of inflammatory prostaglandins. They may be useful in reducing the inflammation and pain that is often associated with IBS. Take three capsules daily.

▸ **Comprehensive digestive enzyme** aids in digestion and can help properly digest foods thus reducing gas and gut tenderness. Include with each meal.

▸ **Soothe and repair the gut** with amino acid L-Glutamine, aloe vera, and herbs such as slippery elm and marshmallow root. Use daily for one month, individually or in combination (see Appendix C).

▸ **Herbal bowel formulas,** which include cascara sagrada, barberry root bark, turkey rhubarb root, support and strengthen colon function. Use when you experience constipation. Avoid harsh laxatives; they can continue to weaken and irritate your gut's lining.

▸ **Ginger tea** can assist in relieving intestinal gas.

▸ **Reduce stress.** Because stress can be a major contributing factor to an irritated gut, find ways to reduce stress, such as journaling, meditation, exercise, and deep breathing.

▸ **Belly breathing** can shift your nervous system into a calm, restorative mode, thereby relaxing a spastic, cramping gut.

▸ **Belly massage** can improve circulation of the blood and lymph and move out trapped gasses and waste matter. Massaging the belly can also help relax muscle spasms, which often accompany IBS. Remember to breathe deeply as you massage.

▸ **Apply warmth** to your abdomen to comfort, soothe, and bring forth blood and nutrients that assist the healing process. Warmth is calming to your nervous system and can help restore proper bowel function. Use a Belly Buddy, hot water bottle, or heating pad.

▸ **Exercise and wisdom-cise stretches** to increase your "feel-good" healing hormones as well as reduce internalized stress.

▸ **Wisdom squat** helps you move out your waste without straining.

▸ **Colon therapy** helps clear out "irritants" and brings quick relief and a clearer awareness to the effects of foe foods on your system.

▶ A **Gut Wisdom Cleanse** rests and assists in the healing process of your digestive and elimination system. It helps you to become aware of cause and effects of your foods. It can often highlight emotions, thoughts, and attitudes that have been bottled within you.

▶ A **comprehensive stool test** may be necessary to check if candida, parasites, or other microorganisms are contributing to your gut's dysfunction (ask your health practitioner or see Appendix C).

▶ **Embrace and conversations with the gut** invites your gut's messages to surface and offers you guidance in your next step of healing.

▶ **Become aware** of who/what is unhealthy in your life. Who or what is irritating you? What toxic emotions are you holding on to? Feel them, express them, and then let them go.

▶ A **forgiveness ceremony** supports your letting go process.

▶ **Thank your gut's wisdom** for causing you enough discomfort that you chose to listen, explore, and make new choices towards healing.

Lactose Intolerance

What Is It?

Sometimes, life just isn't fair. Some people enjoy massive ice cream sundaes, pizza oozing with cheese, and mountainous milk shakes with no problem. Others can put a teaspoon of skim milk in their lattes and suffer gastrointestinal disturbances.

An estimated 50 million Americans and about 70 percent of all adults in the world cannot tolerate milk or dairy products. Lactose intolerance is caused by a deficiency or lack of *lactase,* an enzyme in the small intestine that is responsible for dairy digestion. The lactose (milk sugar) remains undigested, ferments in the colon, and retains fluid, resulting in an ailing belly. The gut begins "speaking" between 30 minutes and a couple of hours after digesting dairy products.

Gut's Wisdom (Symptoms)

- Bloating.
- Abdominal cramping.
- Diarrhea or diarrhea alternating with constipation.
- Mucus and nasal or ear discharge.
- Gas.
- Acne.
- Headaches.
- Nausea.
- Asthma-like reaction (wheezing, rattling cough).

Contributors to Gut Dysfunction: The Gut-Brain Connection

Lactose intolerance occurs in the small intestine. Taoist sages state that the small intestines are like the "officials who are trusted with riches": It is where the "sorting of the pure and impure" occurs. Approximately 90 percent of your nutrients are absorbed into your body for distribution from the small intestine. This relates to more than just food; ideas, beliefs, attitudes, and emotions need to be sorted and the useless discarded. With a lactose intolerance, your gut may be communicating the need for you to allow yourself to receive and "absorb" emotional, mental, and/or spiritual nourishment. You may be being guided to open up, to "take in" and utilize new ideas, beliefs, and so on and let go of unhealthy ones. Because dairy products are associated with nourishment from mother, do you perceive being rejected in certain situations or perhaps are rejecting (most likely unconsciously) love and nurturing being offered to you?

Gut-Brain Attitudes

- Difficulty tolerating and accepting situations.

- Nurturing issues that need to be forgiven and healed.

- Experience difficulty in receiving/taking/digesting new information, experiences, attitudes.

Other Contributors to Gut Dysfunction

▶ Predisposition may often be a root cause. A majority of Asians, African-Americans, and Latinos all genetically lack the ability to digest dairy products efficiently.

▶ Gut disorders such as IBS, celiac disease, or ulcerative colitis may have caused damage to the digestive tract, resulting in impaired dairy digestion.

Befriending Invitations for Creating a Functional Gut

▶ **Refrain from foe foods.** Omit for at least three days, and ideally for 10 days, *all* dairy products. This includes milk, cream, cheese, yogurt, frozen yogurt, and all the sneaky places milk is added: sports bars, lunch meats, cookies, cakes, chocolate, nondairy creamer, and many salad dressings and soups. Be aware of other aliases milk goes by (sodium caseinate, whey, casein, and lactose). After the designated period, slowly bring one or two of the dairy products back into your diet. *Listen to your gut*; it will talk to you loud and clear. If your symptoms return, then dairy is the problem.

▶ **Replace your dairy** with friendly foods such as soy, rice, almond, or Lactaid milk, soy cheese, and rice ice cream. If you eat cheese, use aged hard cheese such as parmesan; it's lower in lactose.

▶ **Use lactase enzymes** when you plan to indulge. You can find these in your local drug or health food store. These supplements will supply you with lactase to help you digest milk sugars.

▶ **Take a calcium supplement.** To be sure you have sufficient calcium in your diet, supplement with a calcium citrate vitamin supplement. Include highly absorbable, nutritious calcium sources such as kale, collard greens, bok choy, spinach, tofu, sardines, calcium-fortified soy milk, apricots, dried figs, almonds, sunflower seeds, cooked dried beans, and yogurt. (Because yogurt is a *fermented* dairy product, many lactose intolerant guts can handle it.)

▶ **Use a dairy-free, refrigerated, high-potency acidophilus capsule or powder,** which will help infuse your gut with lactose-digesting friendly bacteria and promote health digestion. Take two capsules, three times a day or 1 teaspoon of powder in water, twice daily.

▶ **Charcoal tablets** are beneficial for an acute attack when you may have indulged in dairy. It absorbs toxins and gas and relieves diarrhea.

▶ **Apply warmth** in the form of the Belly Buddy or hot water bottle to your abdomen for comfort, nurturing, and relief.

▶ **Belly massage** can assist in moving painful gases out of your system.

▶ **Be aware.** Your gut's wisdom may be guiding you. As you receive new information, "take it in" and put it into practice. Open up to and receive emotional nurturing and nourishment. Make a list of people and situations past and present that you had/have trouble "tolerating." It's time to forgive, embrace, and let go.

▶ **Thank your gut's wisdom** for the guidance it's been sharing with you.

Parasites
What Are They?

A parasite is an organism that lives within or upon another organism, thereby receiving nourishment (parasites get three free meals a day!) at the expense of the host (you). These creepy crawlers are more common that you would imagine. You might think that parasites are a Third World problem or something you can catch only when traveling to the tropics or south-of-the-border countries. Yet parasites can infest and exist in any environment that allows them to survive. In a study of outpatients at the Gastroenterology Clinic in Elmhurst, New York, a 74-percent incidence of parasites was found. A total of 20 percent of this population harbored pathogens. One survey of public health laboratories reported that 15.6 percent of specimens examined contained a parasite. Furthermore, at Great Smokies Diagnostic Laboratory, almost 30 percent of specimens examined are positive for a parasite. Most parasites are microscopic; some others such as pinworms and roundworms are visible to the eye. Parasites mimic other health conditions and often go undiagnosed.

Some parasites excrete toxins causing us to feel toxic, bloated, gassy or nauseous, or just plain "blah." Other parasites damage the gut's lining, leading us to a leaky gut, diarrhea, bloody stools, irritable bowel syndrome, allergies, malabsorption of vitamins and minerals...well, you name it. These guys can throw your whole system out of whack.

More than 20 million Americans have these critters in their gut causing dysfunctions body-wide. If you think you may, too, the truth may make you feel miserable at first but, remember: It will set you free!

Gut's Wisdom (Symptoms)

- Fatigue (chronic).
- Itching anus.
- Rashes.
- IBS.
- Chronic diarrhea or constipation.
- Bloody stools.
- Abdominal cramping.
- Sleep disturbances.
- Teeth grinding.

- Poor immune system.
- Allergies/food sensitivities.
- Sugar cravings.
- Joint and muscle aches.
- Unexplained weight loss.
- Unexplained fever.
- Persistent skin problems.
- Anemia.
- Prostatitis.
- Irritability/nervousness.

Contributors to Gut Dysfunction: The Gut-Brain Connection

Parasites feed off you, often damaging the protective lining of your gut as they deviate mental and physical health. Are you unable to say "no"? Do you lack personal boundaries? Do you feel that someone "sucks" off of you and drains you? In what situations do you feel like a victim or feel that you've lost your center or inner power? In what ways do you leave yourself open and vulnerable to outside negative influences that come in, invade, or rob your mental, emotional, or spiritual vitality?

Gut-Brain Attitudes

- Giving power to others in your life.
- Feeling like a victim.

- Having weak personal boundaries.
- Being vulnerable or sensitive to outside negative influences.

Other Contributors to Gut Dysfunction

▶ **Water** is one of the primary sources of parasitic infection. Drinking unfiltered water from streams, lakes, or rivers, or even swimming in lakes and rivers, can expose you to parasites. Our tap water can also be a carrier. In 1993, Milwaukee's water supply was contaminated with an outbreak of Cryptosporidium (a microscopic parasite). This outbreak made 400,000 people ill and killed 40.

▶ **Foods** at home or in restaurants that have not been thoroughly cleaned or have been handled by those with unwashed hands.

▶ **Poor digestion** due to a lack of proper digestive enzymes, particularly hydrochloric acid, which is produced in your stomach to digest protein and kill unwanted invaders. Remember that *antacids* inhibit this function in your stomach.

▶ **Antibiotic use** destroys your protective gut bacteria, leaving you vulnerable for unfriendly critters.

▶ **Over-consumption of foe sugars and refined carbohydrates** can affect the balance of your protective friendly bacteria, allowing parasites to flourish. (Some parasites are sugar-lovers.)

▶ **Pets.** Yes, your "best friend" can often transmit parasites to you. Dogs, cats, and birds are self-groomers and can pass "waste" bacteria and parasites to you.

▶ **Traveling** outside the United States, especially to underdeveloped countries, can expose you to parasites. Bear in mind that folks in the United States also have our fair share. Remember that many of our foods are imported from south of the border.

▶ **If you are in contact** with someone who has parasites (a carrier), they can be transmitted to you.

▶ **Raw fish (sushi), steak tartare, and pork** can be contaminated and carry parasites.

Befriending Inoitations for Creating a Functional Gut

Ask your health practitioner for a **Comprehensive Digestive Stool Analysis (CDSA)** with a parasitology test to assess if parasites are the reason your gut has been speaking to you (see Appendix C). This particular test can identify the "critter(s)" and give you specific guidelines for treatment, whether through herbal preparations or prescription medications. Note: Medical parasite testing generally only detects approximately 20 percent of parasites. If you suspect parasites, you may choose to forgo the testing and embark on a 90-day herbal program to put a demise to these critters.

▶ **Clear** is a powerful antiparasitic herbal combination that includes black walnut, black seed, cloves, cramp bark, fennel seed, hyssop, pumpkin seed, peppermint leaves, gentian root, thyme, and grapefruit seed. This formula has been extremely beneficial in eradicating parasites and the accompanying symptoms. It is used for a 90-day period for a successful outcome. Because parasite larvae have a hatching cycle, you want to make sure you have eradicated these tenacious critters. (See Appendix C to order.)

Additionally, raw garlic, pumpkin seed, and black walnut tincture have been traditionally used for their anti-parasitic properties.

▶ **Anti-parasite medications** may be needed and are sometimes the most efficient approach, because the parasites can burrow themselves into the intestinal wall. Note: These medications can be quite disruptive to your liver and intestinal bacteria, so take care and replenish friendly bacteria.

▶ **Acidophilus and bifidus** are the friendly gut bacteria, which need to be replenished within your gut during and after herbal or prescription medications. Recommended usage: Take two capsules, three times a day or 1 teaspoon of powder in water, twice daily.

▶ **Enhance digestion with a digestive aid** that includes hydrochloric acid, which helps kill parasites when or if they enter your digestive system. Take as directed with each meal.

▶ **Follow Gut Wisdom friendly food choices** to maintain a healthy alkaline pH balance, because acidity invites parasites.

▶ **Glutamine (an amino acid), deglycyrrhizinated licorice, or aloe vera concentrate, slippery elm, and marshmallow root herbs** help repair the intestinal mucous lining, which is often damaged due to parasites making themselves at home within your body. Recommended usage: 1/2 teaspoon, three times a day for three months.

▶ A **Gut Wisdom Cleanse** helps clear out parasites and prevent reabsorbtion of their toxic by-products into your system.

▶ **Colon therapy** is very important to keep your gut clear, because parasites burrow into the excessive mucous lining of the intestinal tract. Colonics will also flush out parasites that have died off with your parasite cleanse. Symptoms occurring from parasite die-off can be minimized significantly.

▶ **Belly breathing** helps restore relaxation and proper bowel functioning.

▶ **Warmth on your abdomen** with a Belly Buddy or hot water bottle restores good digestion and elimination.

▶ **Travel.** (See "Traveling With Your Bowels" on page 223.)

▶ **Prevention.** Keep your bowels healthy and moving. Carefully wash all fruit and vegetables. Wash your hands especially after petting your "best friend." Think twice about eating raw fish (sushi). Keep your immune system strong; this is your best defense.

▶ **Be aware of attitudes and outside influences** that disempower you. Set clear boundaries; learn to say no. Let go of people and situations that are "sucking" energy from you. *Take back your power!*

▶ **Thank your gut** for being the messenger for you to make some important empowering dietary and attitude shifts.

Ulcer

What Is It?

Approximately 14 million Americans have suffered or are suffering from an ulcer. An ulcer is an open sore in the lining of your stomach (*gastric ulcer*) or your duodenum, which is the first part of your small intestine (*duodenal ulcer*). The tissue surrounding the ulcer is generally irritated and inflamed.

Generally, we have a mucous layer protecting our stomach's tissue from being gnawed away by our own gastric secretions (pepsin, hydrochloric acid). If there is an excess of stomach acid or the protective mucus isn't replaced due to our gut troublemakers, an ulcer is a possible outcome. The bacteria of Helicobacter pylori has been also implicated. An untreated ulcer can cause bleeding into your intestinal tract and is an extremely serious conditional that can be fatal. Gastritis is an inflammation of the stomach lining—but without a sore or ulcer. Nevertheless, it should be attended to with the same concern as an ulcer.

Gut's Wisdom (Symptoms)

- Chronic abdominal burning.
- Gnawing abdominal pain after eating (stomach ulcer).
- Gnawing abdominal pain two to three hours after eating (duodenal ulcer).
- Pain subsides with food, drinking water, or taking antacids.
- Nausea.
- Diarrhea.
- Vomiting.

Contributors to Gut Dysfunction: The Gut-Brain Connection

The stomach is the primary organ for storing, diluting, and digesting food. It is a symbol of the thoughts, ideas, and inspiration that we digest and assimilate.

Stomach "challenges" such as an ulcer often reflect how we "take in" or digest life's experiences. According to the insights and wisdom of Louise Hay, author of *You Can Heal Your Life,* ulcers are a result of holding and feelings of *fear.* Fear can show up as thoughts and feelings of not being good enough as a parent, employee, boss, spouse, lover, or friend. Hay suggests that, by feeding these feelings of fear, "we rip our guts apart trying to please others."

At some level and in different ways, we are concerned about how we look in the eyes of others. This is why we push for deadlines, repress aggressive feelings, and so on and why we end up feeling raw and exposed and with internal pain.

Are there unexpressed aggravations and/or old memories burning you up inside? What is eating away at you? Can you allow yourself to "just be" and not be a human doer? What feelings need to be expressed and released?

Gut-Brain Attitudes

- Worry.
- Anxiety.
- Fear.
- Obsessing.
- Repressed feelings.
- Time/deadline pressures.
- Feeling raw and exposed.
- A person who/experience that is constantly irritating you.
- Concerns of not being good enough.

Other Contributors to Gut Dysfunction: The Gut-Brain Connection

▸ **Medications** such as nonsteroidal anti-inflammatory drugs (NSAIDs), steroids, aspirin, Motrin, Advil, and Tylenol are contributors to approximately 10 percent of duodenal and stomach ulcers.

▸ **Foe foods** such as refined sugar and flour products (cookies, cakes), red meat, fried foods, alcohol, soft drinks, and coffee can all contribute to gut (stomach and duodenal) irritations, which can eventually lead to ulcers.

▸ **Alcohol and coffee (even decaffeinated)** stimulate excessive stomach acid secretions.

▸ **Smoking** can contribute to ulcers as well as compromise your gut's healing ability. "It may stunt its healing, and contribute to recurrence," says Dr. R. Hoffman, author of *Seven Weeks to a Settled Stomach.* "Smoking inhibits prostaglandin production which is a 'care taker' hormone that makes sure your stomach lining is protected."

▸ **Antacids** can exacerbate ulcer formation. According to Dr. R. Hoffman's *Seven Weeks to a Settled Stomach*, some popular antacids contain aspirin, so large doses of these drugs may even *cause* ulcers instead of soothe them. Another common antacid ingredient, calcium carbonate, actually *stimulates* increased gastric secretion!

▸ **Ulcer drugs** such as Tagamet or Zantac block production of stomach acid and may suppress your symptoms, but seldom is the ulcer healed. On top of that, with no stomach acid available, protein cannot be digested properly, which means that putrefaction and gas occur. Harmful bacteria and other undesirable microorganisms from your daily food ingestion are not killed off, leaving your gut vulnerable.

▸ **Helicobacter pylori (H-pylori)** is a bacteria found between the stomach lining and mucous membrane. Research has shown that a majority of those who have ulcers have this bacteria. It is believed that those with poor lifestyle choices and stress, which can compromise the immune system, may be more susceptible to the H-pylori taking hold in their guts.

▸ **Constant worry, anxiety, fear, and stress** may increase the production of stomach acid, leaving you susceptible to ulcer formation.

Befriending Invitations for Creating a Functional Gut

▶ **Medical test for H-pylori.** If you test positive, the doctor may treat you with antibiotics, bismuth (protects stomach lining), and/or an anti-parasitic.

▶ **Wise dietary and lifestyle revisions.** Omit sugar, coffee and tea (even decaf), soft drinks, alcohol, spicy food, red meat, refined foods, fatty foods, and milk. All can cause an increase in stomach acid secretion. Omit or cut back on smoking, steroid medications, and NSAIDs (if possible), aspirin, and antacids.

▶ **Eat more fiber.** Research has found a connection between a low-fiber diet and the occurrence and development of ulcers. Fiber increases the movement of toxins and bacteria through the digestive and eliminative systems, leaving less time for bacterial invasion. So, possibly, fiber may not give H-pylori an opportunity to make a home in your gut—no squatters allowed! Fiber and fiber-rich foods help promote the secretion of mucin, which aids in protecting against ulcer formation. Ground flax seed mixed with juice or in your cereal (one to two tablespoons) has a buffering and healing effect on excess acid and is soothing for your inflamed belly. Rice and millet are high-fiber grains that are gentle on your ulcerated gut. Plenty of green vegetables contain vitamin K (needed for healing). Eating steamed veggies is easier on a sensitive gut. If symptoms are severe, pulverize them like baby food in a blender.

▶ **Plain yogurt** can soothe as well as supply your gut with healing friendly bacteria.

▶ **Baked or broiled fish, chicken, turkey, or tofu** generally is easier to digest than red meat.

▶ **Fruits.** Bananas seem to be the kindest to an ulcerated gut.

▶ **Water** can reduce the pain of an ulcer flare-up. When in pain, drink four to six glasses of water at room temperature.

▶ **Check for food allergies/sensitivities.** Any additional irritation may slow down the healing process. Many nutritionists believe food allergies or sensitivities are a prime contributing cause to ulcers.

▶ **Chew your food** thoroughly to assist your gut in proper digestion.

▶ **Eat small meals** throughout the day.

▶ **Use Wisdom Food Combining** to ease digestibility and absorption; this is a good way to be gentle to your gut and reduce further irritation.

Repair and Soothe Your Stomach Lining

▶ **L-glutamine** is significant in supporting the healing of peptic ulcers. Suggested use is 500 mg daily on an empty stomach.

▶ **Flax seed oil** is an essential fatty acid used to increase prostaglandin production that promotes repair and healing and regulates inflammation. Suggested use is two capsules, three times daily.

▶ **Licorice DGL (deglycyrrhized)** promotes healing of gastric and duodenal ulcers by increasing prostaglandins that support stomach cell repair and reduce inflammation. Follow directions on label. *Do not* substitute ordinary licorice or licorice candy; they do not have the same effect. Use as directed.

▶ **Aloe vera juice** aids in relief of pain and enhances healing. Take 4 ounces daily.

▶ **Acidophilus and bifidus** are gut protectors and keep friendly bacteria abundant for continued protection and healing. Recommended use is two capsules, three times daily.

▶ **Liquid chlorophyll** has soothing and healing properties. Follow directions on the bottle.

▶ **Slippery elm and marshmallow herbs** help heal mucous membranes and gut inflamed tissue. Drink 3 cups daily.

▶ **Goldenseal** is also very healing and soothing to your mucous membranes and enhances immune function. It is easiest to take in capsule form (it is a bit bitter). Take three capsules, three times a day, for up to three months.

▶ **Multivitamins and minerals** include nutrients that support a stronger immune system, thereby enhancing your ability to heal. It is suggested that you include them daily with your meals.

▶ **Ulcer-healer juice** is a freshly made juice of cabbage that has a rich supply of calcium and chlorophyll—both necessary for overall repairing and rebuilding. To make it more palatable, combine it with celery, parsley, and apple.

▶ **Stress-reducing juice** is a freshly made juice of lettuce, carrots, tomato, and celery that helps calm frazzled nerves. Drink at least one 8-ounce glass daily.

▶ **Belly breathing** helps you to relax, reduce stress and anxiety. Each breath brings oxygen into your cells to assist healing.

▸ **Warmth** is very calming for a stressed gut (and person). Use a Belly Buddy or hot water bottle to bring comfort and a supply of blood and nutrients for healing this tender area.

▸ A **Gut Wisdom Cleanse** can give your gut a rest and time to heal. It allows you to discern the cause and effect of your foods have on your stomach ailment.

▸ **Embracing and conversation with the gut.** Important tools you can use to comfort an irritated stomach and receive guidance to assist your healing.

▸ **Movement** is a wonderful way to release your internalized stress.

▸ **Wisdom Journaling** gets stressful thoughts and emotions down on paper and out of you!

▸ **Be aware;** take time to be nourished. As they say, "Let go and let God." Worry begets more worry. Attend to attitudes that lead you to believe you have to do it all by a certain time and all in the right way. Let go of the attitude, person, and/or situation that is "eating you up" inside. Prayer, meditation, and good counseling can assist you in this journey.

▸ **Thank your gut** for the messages and wisdom.

Colon Cancer
What Is It?

The word *cancer* puts the fear of God in many of us. The fact is, if it is detected early enough, it is often preventable, as well as treatable. According to the American Cancer Society, colon and colorectal cancer are the second leading causes of death due to cancer. It is second only to lung cancer. More than 130,000 Americans will be diagnosed this year. The majority of those diagnosed will be 50 years of age and older. Approximately 60,000 will not survive. The Cancer Research Foundation states that if colorectal cancer is detected in its earliest stage, it is more than 90 percent curable.

Cancer is a mutation of healthy cells. As cell division occurs within the colon the DNA uncoils, predisposing a large surface for possible damage. During cell division there is less energy available to protect and repair the DNA. Therefore it becomes vulnerable to unhealthy exposure and errors, such as cell mutations that alter genetic information. Polyps are a form of this mutation.

The majority of colorectal cancer begins as polyps, growths in the lining of the colon or rectum. Most polyps are small, benign growths and can be detected and removed. However, if undetected and untreated, a percentage of polyps keeps growing and mutating until they transform into cancerous tumors and burrow deep into the muscle wall that surrounds the colon. The cancer cells can spread into the blood and lymph systems to other areas of the body and continue reproducing. Cancer cells are not receptive to the normal signals to stop reproducing and may affect other organs and their functions.

There are a few rare types of colon cancers (accounting for 1 to 5 percent) that do not occur from polyps: hereditary nonpolyposis colorectal cancer (HNPCC) and adenomatous polyposis. There is ongoing research trying to determine why these cells take on a life of their own. We do know that there are certain risk factors that increase the likelihood of cancer developing. Free radicals are potentially carcinogenic substances that form through the body's metabolism and reproduce faster if unhealthy eating habits, environmental contaminants, and stress are present and are able to impair the immune system. This has been considered to be a significant factor in the contribution of uncontrolled cellular growth.

Gut's Wisdom (Symptoms)

- Change in bowel habits.
- Blood in stool or black stool (bowel movement).
- Abdominal cramps.
- Changes in stool consistency.
- Jet black stools.
- Unusual weight loss.
- Chronic abdominal pain.
- Fatigue/anemia (due to bleeding).
- Persistent abdominal pain.

If you have any of these symptoms or a combination, please get to a doctor and get tested NOW!

Contributors to Gut Dysfunction: The Gut-Brain Connection

The colon and rectum are associated with the "letting go" process of waste that is no longer beneficial—both digested food waste *and* emotional waste. Holding on to long-felt repressed or unexpressed attitudes and feelings create internalized stress, which is both toxic internally as well as externally. Internally these stresses poison us and inhibit our gut function and immune system. Holding on distorts and mutates how we perceive our present moments and how we view our life and possibly taint it with regrets, grief, anger, despair, and resentment toward ourselves and others. When the natural defensive action of the immune system is weakened, the potential of abnormal body cells taking over can develop. These abnormal cells behave differently from the others. They often become isolated (a tumor) and/or spread, undermining the survival of the whole being.

Be aware and examine. Are you cut off and isolated from your feelings? Do you suppress or ignore your feelings; do you bury traumas or deny your own needs for the sake of others? Do you experience a sense of powerlessness or defensiveness when confronted with a person perceived as stronger, leaving you feeling overpowered or worthless? All of these circumstances ignore the healthy emotional nourishment of your whole being.

Gut-Brain Attitudes

- Holding on to past anger, resentment, grief.
- Unforgiving of self.
- A "wanting to give up" attitude.
- Self-hatred.
- A deep emotional hurt eating away at you.

Other Contributors to Gut Dysfunction

▸ **Physical and emotional stress** releases adrenaline and cortisol within our bodies, and our fight-or-flight response kicks in. Cortisol is a powerful immuno-suppresant. High levels of cortisol are associated with cancer. In *Eat Right or Die Young,* Dr. Cass Igram states that "grief, distress, fear, worry and anger are emotions which have horrible effects on the body's function. Researchers have discovered that these emotions cause the release of chemicals—neuropeptides. These potent compounds have a profound immune-suppressive action. Scientists have traced a pathway from the brain to the immune cells proving that negative emotions can stop the immune cells dead in their track.... Once this happens, harmful microbes or cancer cells can invade any tissue in the body."

▸ **Genetic predispositions.** A family history of colon and/or ovarian, bladder, or prostate cancers increases the risk of colon cancer.

▸ **High-fat/low-fiber factors.** Substantial research links a high-fat/low-fiber diet to cancer (cheese, red meat, eggs, fried foods, and hydrogenated fats). High-fat diets stimulate the metabolism and consequently will create an excessive amount of bile, which will be released via the liver into the colon. Bile contains the toxins and cancer-causing chemicals (preservatives, pesticides, hormone by-products) that your body is attempting to move out through the colon. Without fiber, these toxins will not be able to move! The longer waste material remains in the colon, the more concentrated the bile acids become, irritating the colon lining. Americans generally eat about 12 grams of fiber daily, compared to the National Cancer Institute's daily recommended 20 to 30 grams.

▶ **Foe foods** offer little nutritional value to strengthen our bodies. We, then, compromise the liver and pancreas to produce extra enzymes to attempt to digest these foods. As these organs are over-taxed, our immune system is compromised.

▶ **Ulcerative colitis and inflammatory bowel disorder (IBD)** involve an inflammation of part of the digestive tract. Symptoms of IBD can include anemia, abdominal cramps, and bloody and mucus-filled diarrhea. There is a higher incidence of colon cancer in individuals who suffer from ulcerative colitis

▶ **Low butyric acid levels.** Butyric acid is a short-chain fatty acid, created from friendly bacteria and fiber that is used to nourish the cells of the intestines for the purpose of regeneration and protection. Inhibited butyric acid levels have been associated with ulcerative colitis and colon cancer.

▶ **Heavy alcohol consumption** may compromise the body's immune system by depleting our precious vitamin and mineral supply. In addition, food choices are generally inadequate when alcohol is running the show.

▶ **Free radicals** are potentially carcinogenic substances that form in your body via your own metabolism. They are created under certain conditions such as smoking, environmental pollution, chemicals in our foods and household items, poor diet, illnesses, and our old friend stress.

▶ **Gut imbalances** such as dybosis (an imbalance between bad, toxic bacteria and friendly, protective bacteria) contribute to putrefaction in the gut. These putrefactive bacteria are not carcinogenic by themselves, but when they are in contact with bile acids they become potential tumor-promoters.

▶ **Lack of exercise** allows toxins and carcinogens to linger due to sluggish bowel function. A "couch potato" tends to be oxygen-deprived, and research suggests that cancer cells tend to live in an oxygen-depleted environment.

Befriending Invitations for Creating a Functional Gut

▶ **Early detection and prevention.** When colon cancer is detected early, it is a highly treatable disease. (See Appendix B for information about early-detection tests.) The screening recommendation for colorectal cancer and polyps is to begin screening at age 50. But if there is a family history or personal history of colon cancers, other cancers, polyps, ulcerated colitis (reoccurring inflammation of the lining of the colon), or Crohn's (recurring inflammation of the intestines that can cause damage which penetrates all layers of the colon), or if your gut is voicing suspicious symptoms, it is recommended that you listen to your gut and have a screening sooner. Taking proactive, preventive measures is the wisest choice. It's impossible to avoid all of the risk factors of developing cancer, but you can reduce your odds with prevention choices.

▶ **A strong immune system** is critical to prevention, especially from an opportunistic disease such as cancer. So, to build a strong immune system:

> ⊳ **The Gut Wisdom Diet is a low-fat/high-fiber diet** with an abundance of vegetables, fruits, whole grains, and high-quality proteins. Supplement with 2 to 3 tablespoons of ground flax seed daily to ensure adequate fiber intake. Flax seed is the richest known source of lignans, which have anti-carcinogenic properties. Remember: Fiber binds potentially carcinogenic compounds, as well as other harmful toxins and gut irritants, and swiftly moves them out of your colon. Eat up!

> ⊳ **Reduce or omit alcohol.** It's time to find another activity, one that enhances your immune system.

> ⊳ **Protective bacteria**, acidophilus and bifidus, are musts in order to prevent putrefaction. Putrefaction leads to an imbalance of friendly, protective bacteria and unfriendly, harmful ones. Your gut is no longer protected from the increase of toxic, possibly cancer-causing substances. Numerous studies and research on the effects and role of friendly bacteria as a cancer fighter and protector have been documented. According to the article "The Role of Diet [fermented dairy—acidophilus] in the Causation and Prevention of Cancer" by Barry R. Golen of Tufts University of Medicine, published in *The Causation and Prevention of Cancer* (1989), friendly bacteria is a cancer-fighter and protector.

> **Greens and more greens.** Green vegetable juices are power-ful detoxifiers as well as a source of cleansing and immune-system-boosting chlorophyll, minerals, and enzymes. A mixture of spinach, broccoli, parsley, and carrots is a powerful combination. Pick up a juicer and juice cookbook and try different combinations. Wheat grass, barley green, chlorella, chlorophyll, and alfalfa are cancer-fighting nutrients. They can be found in tablet and powder form. Wheat grass is best when taken in fresh juice form or straight up. Check out your local health food stores or juice bar. There are healing retreats and fasting centers that focus heavily on using "greens" for prevention and assisting healing. Healing miracles occur (see Appendix C)!

> **Green tea** has anti-cancer properties. It is an immune-system stimulator and combats free radical damage. Recent research in Japan shows that green tea reduces cancer-related death rates.

> **Digestive enzymes** make certain that you digest and assimilate the friendly foods you are eating in order to keep your immune system strong. They should be taken with each meal.

> **Vitamins C, A, and E and selenium** can help protect cells from potentially carcinogenic free radicals. Vitamin B complex is necessary for normal cell division and function. A comprehensive multivitamin and mineral tablet taken daily is recommended.

> **Folic acid** protects cells from mutating and turning cancerous. Enjoy and ingest folic acid-rich foods such as asparagus, leafy vegetables, fish, sunflower seeds, or citrus fruits. Recommended daily usage is 400 milligrams.

> **Calcium** is presently being researched for polyp prevention, as it may keep cells from proliferating. Supplement with calcium citrate daily (use as directed) and/or eat calcium-rich foods such as beans, broccoli, collard greens, kale, almonds, sunflower seeds, and yogurt.

> **Flax seed oil** is rich in lignans, which research has suggested plays a key role in the prevention of colon cancer. It is a source of omega-3, an essential acid that works on the cellular level to reduce and prevent inflammation. Recommended usage is 1 teaspoon daily.

▷ **Minimize environmental toxins.** You may not have control over the quality of the air you breath, but you do have control over the water you drink, the cleaning supplies you use, the foods you purchase and eat, and the cigarettes you (don't!) smoke. So drink only purified water, use air purifiers, use nontoxic, biodegradable cleaning supplies, eat organic foods, and *don't* smoke!

▷ **Keep your colon moving.** Do a Gut Wisdom three- or seven-day cleanse biyearly and/or do short, one-day Gut Wisdom cleanses each month, and get colonics/enemas. Cleansing the liver and colon has immeasurable benefits of keeping you free of potentially toxic, carcinogenic substances and strengthening your immune system.

▷ **Movement, exercise, and wisdom-cise stretches** release immune-enhancing chemicals. Increased blood circulation enhances nourishment and cleansing of body tissues. Exercise brings oxygen into your tissues. Some research suggests that the more oxygen in the bloodstream, the less opportunity cancer has to survive. In addition, exercise burns fat. Many cancers are related to fat-soluble toxins. The less fat on your body, the less fat-soluble toxins your body can store.

▷ **Belly breathing** gives you and your gut a destressing. Belly breathing also boosts the immune system. It activates the calming and restorative function of the parasympathetic nervous system.

▷ **Embrace and conversations with the gut** encourage a relationship dialogue with your gut's wisdom. They invite you to explore the message and provide guidance of what you need to do to support healing. Compassion and clarity have the ability to change the biochemistry of your gut and body.

▷ **Warmth on the belly** is comforting and stress-reducing and helps restore proper digestive and eliminative function. Use a Belly Buddy or hot water bottle daily.

▷ A **forgiveness ceremony** assists you in letting go and forgiving yourself and others. When anger and resentment are released, there is room for joy and love. Love enhances the immune system.

▷ **Thank your gut** for the messages that could save your life, and thank yourself for following through.

> ▷ **Open up** to support and connection with others. Feel, express, and release pent-up emotions. Journal or receive guidance from qualified therapists to help you move through painful experiences in order to let go. Be diligent but gentle with yourself.

Traveling With Your Bowels

What Is It?

Don't worry—they won't leave home without you, though sometimes you may wish they would! Many of us love traveling but have *bowel reservations*: the fear of getting constipated or having loose bowels, troubles that make a potentially wonderful trip uncomfortable, at best, and *horrible, at worst*!

Prior to or during one's travels, a doctor may prescribe an antibiotic as a prophylactic to prevent infection by harmful bacteria. Many people choose to pop antacids due to the no-holds-barred vacation food fest, and many others take prescription medications. As you have learned from reading this book, all of these set the gut up for an attack by unruly and opportunistic bacteria. Antibiotics, antacids, and medications all throw off the balance of delicate, friendly bacteria. Once the balance is upset, everything is invited into the gut to live, ruining a good vacation and a pleasant homecoming.

Contributors to Gut Dysfunction: The Gut-Brain Connection

▶ Montezuma's revenge. Travelers' diarrhea may occur as you are enjoying the foods and libations in South America, Asia, or Africa that were contaminated with the intestinal bacteria E-coli, salmonella, or campylobacter (although these intestinal bacteria can, in fact, be acquired anywhere). Montezuma will generally run its course and you will probably be fine once you get home. However, if you've acquired a parasite (for example, Giardia lamblia), you will continue to have diarrhea plus other persistent gut symptoms (see the "Parasites" section in this chapter) until some aggressive action involving prescription medication is taken.

▶ Drinking contaminated water that can be filled with undesirable organisms. Many countries lack strict standards for water filtration.

▶ Eating contaminated foods. In some countries the water used to grow as well as wash foods may be contaminated with inadequately filtered water. Dairy products may be unpasteurized and possibly contain harmful strains of bacteria.

▸ Overindulging with reckless abandon with beverages and foods taxes your digestive and elimination systems, resulting in undesirable gut ailments.

▸ Anxiety and stress of flying, leaving your home, children, and so forth. (Even the excitement of leaving can be stressful.) This inhibits proper gut function leaving you with indigestion, constipation, and/or diarrhea.

Befriending Invitations for Creating a Functional Gut

Preparing your gut for traveling:

▸ **Acidophilus and bifidus** can be prophylactic gut protection. Recommendation: If you are not presently taking these supplements, begin with two capsules, three times daily, two weeks prior to your trip.

▸ **Digestive enzymes** are powerful protection against undesirable bacteria taking hold. Enzymes will help kill the "undesirables" before they can begin to cause gut voices of discomfort within you. Recommendation: Begin or continue supplementing with each meal. (Avoid a digestive enzyme that includes hydrochloric acid if you suspect or have been diagnosed with an ulcer.)

▸ **Boost your immune system** to guard your system against bacteria in airplanes, food, and water. Recommendation: Two weeks prior to your trip, include the immune enhancing herb echinacea. Use as directed.

▸ **Belly breathing** supports good bowel functions. Nobody likes to breathe deeply on an airplane, but you can still belly breathe by using a tissue with a little lavender oil (known for its calming affect) on it. This will help reduce the stress of flying, which results in inhibited gut function. Avoid (as much as possible) the food served on planes or in airports.

▸ **Bring your own snacks:** fruit, nuts, dried mixed fruit, and rice cakes. *Drink plenty of bottled water to keep your bowels hydrated.*

Survival Pack for Traveling Bowels

You won't need another suitcase for the following. This gut vacation survival pack can be put in baggies for the length of your stay.

▸ **LBC-Lax and cascara sagrada** are gentle, natural, herbal bowel laxatives.

▸ **Super Green tablets** can be a source of fiber and nutrients, as your diet selections during your travels may not be vegetables. Recommendation: Four to six capsules daily.

▶ **Metamucil or ground flax seed** is easy to mix in a hotel room. Take it in the morning and in the evening. Always follow with a full glass of purified, bottled water.

▶ Include **digestive enzymes and acidophilus/bifidus** with each meal. This will eliminate the need for antacids, reduce gas, and kill "foreigner" bacteria before it makes itself at home.

▶ **Ginger capsules or tea** can be used for motion sickness, which will help minimize nausea.

▶ **Wisdom squat** at the toilet. Use a foot stool (or the waste paper basket or thick telephone book) at the base of the toilet to help assist an easy bowel movement.

▶ **Belly breathe** to release the anxiety. Thinking that you may not be able to eliminate just tightens your gut even more.

▶ **Suppositories** can be helpful to activate a bowel movement. Recommendation: vitamin E or tea tree oil suppositories.

When Diarrhea Hits

▶ Use **charcoal capsules** every two hours until diarrhea subsides.

▶ **Pepto-Bismol** can help clear diarrhea with no side effects, however your stool will be black due to the bismuth. **Imodium A-D** slows down your peristalsis (bowel muscle contraction) thus allowing your waste to absorb more water. **Kaopectate** bulks up your waste and may help absorb as well as trap bacteria. **Bentonite** is a volcanic ash that absorbs 10 times its weight. It will grab and hold on to bacteria to eventually move it out of your system.

▶ **Eat lightly when diarrhea speaks.** Choose white rice, bananas, applesauce, and herbal teas (not exactly vacation food).

Enjoy your travels.

Getting Off Laxatives

Laxatives are common remedies for constipation. According to the American Cancer Association, more than 20 million Americans are laxative users. Used occasionally, most laxatives will help you move out what seems to be stuck within. However, millions of people are *dependent* on the assistance of laxatives, and the mere thought of life without them brings fear and a tightened gut—which just makes them want to just pop another laxative!

More often than not, laxatives are overused by people who are uncomfortable and frustrated with their constipated guts. Overuse of laxatives weaken bowel muscles; eventually even the strongest pill will no longer work.

Although I sympathize with the desire to get that waste out, I encourage options that honor and heal the gut. Let me suggest some safer options.

Contributors to Gut Dysfunction: The Gut-Brain Connection

▶ **Foe foods** you are sensitive or allergic to, lactose intolerance, and inadequate fiber and water can all keep you stuck and dependent on laxatives.

▶ **Medications** can slow intestinal muscular function or dehydrate the bowel contents.

▶ **Avoiding the call of Mother Nature** when she is giving you obvious signals to let go can teach your gut to become lazy.

▶ **The abuse of laxatives** creates a dependency on the pill rather than listening to what your guts needs.

▶ **Dybosis,** an imbalance of friendly versus unfriendly gut bacteria, results in a malfunctioning colon.

▶ **Couch Potato Syndrome** can result in a couch-potato colon—that is, one that's not moving.

▶ **Stress** inhibits proper gut function.

▶ **Emotional "holding on"** to feelings, attitudes, and beliefs can and often do manifest as a physical holding on.

Befriending Invitations for Creating a Functional Gut

▶ **Gut Wisdom Diet and supplements** support proper gut function. It is rich in fiber and low in foe fat. Include extra fiber daily by including 2 to 3 tablespoons of ground flax seeds mixed in juice or cereals.

▶ **Acidophilus and bifidus** regulate bowel peristalsis. Recommendation: Two capsules, three times daily.

▶ **Omega-3 oils** to keep the colon lubricated, healed, and moving efficiently. Recommendation: Three capsules daily.

▶ **Digestive enzymes** will assist in the proper digestion of food, which will avoid gut irritations and inflammations, minimizing constipation. Recommendation: Use with each meal.

▸ **Super Green tablets or capsules** are an excellent source of extra fiber. If you find eating sufficient vegetables daily a challenge, using Green supplements is extremely beneficial. Recommendation: Use a product that contains wheat grass, alfalfa, barley grass, spirulina. Use individually or in combination. Use as suggested.

▸ **Medications** you may use daily can cause constipation. Discuss this with your doctor.

▸ **Cascara sagrada** or other natural herbal bowel supplements are safe and natural herbal laxatives and can be used to strengthen and tone weakened bowels and wean yourself off of harsher, chemical laxatives. Begin with one capsule at each meal and increase as needed. As your gut gets stronger and the bowels begin operating more efficiently, you can decrease the intake of these herbal tablets.

▸ **Vitamin C** taken in higher doses can help soften stool. Increase daily to determine your daily needs.

▸ **Magnesium** enhances bowel tone, which helps keep your bowel peristalsis working. Suggested 400 milligrams daily.

▸ **Get juiced.** Ideally, a daily glass of a green vegetable juice will enhance bowel function.

▸ **Train your bowels.** Make it a habit to sit on the toilet every morning for 10 minutes. Don't ignore Mother Nature when she knocks; go directly to the restroom.

▸ **Wisdom squatting** helps by alleviating excessive straining, allowing the lower portion of the bowel to be stimulated and thus activate a bowel movement. Use a foot stool at the base of the toilet and place your feet on it to simulate a squatting posture. Belly breathe, relax, and place warmth (Belly Buddy or hot water bottle) on your abdomen with the intention of "letting go."

▸ **Hot and cold water flush** directly on your belly each day to help stimulate its function.

▸ **Gut Wisdom Cleanse** will assist in getting your gut on track and help you detect the foe foods that may be contributing to a sluggish bowel.

▸ **Colon therapy** helps strengthen the peristaltic action (the colon's natural rhythmic muscle relaxation and contraction) and clears and frees the gut of accumulated waste matter that may be inhibiting proper bowel function. Also, once the gut is cleared, one is much more aware of what foods slow your bowel function down, allowing for greater body-gut awareness. Colon therapy is beneficial when one is weaning oneself off of laxatives and making dietary and/or lifestyle changes.

▸ **Let go;** journal all the "toxic" thoughts, attitudes, and beliefs you have been holding onto. Free yourself and your gut.

▸ **Embrace and converse with your gut** to comfort, listen, and explore what your gut needs. This process can help you gain insight into what you have been holding on to.

▸ **Thank your gut wisdom for this valuable, sometimes uncomfortable, inner journey of healing.**

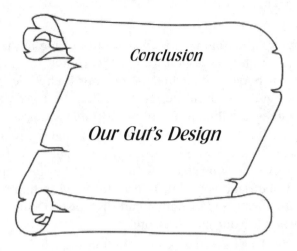

Conclusion

Our Gut's Design

I was having dinner with a few acquaintances and was asked to describe this book project. As is any author, I was eager to talk about my work, but I couldn't help but notice the surprised looks I was getting as I waxed on about the discomforts and dangers of autointoxication and the effects our poor food choices, thoughts, and attitudes have on our gut's health.

"I just can't believe it," said Elaine, one of my dinner companions. "I thought our bodies are designed to process all the different kinds of foods we eat and handle our daily stresses. Is it really such a problem?"

No matter how beautifully our bodies were designed, they weren't designed for the modern, Western world. Our bodies haven't changed all that much from the time the first Homo sapiens walked the Earth. They were built to digest whole grains and vegetables and the occasional bit of meat, not the nearly *200 pounds* of meat the average American consumes per year. We weren't designed to process cups of coffee the size of flower pots that artificially stimulate the bowel to frantic, inefficient activity. Our ancestors didn't drop by the nearest McDonald's or Wendy's for huge, fat-laden meals that tax the gut and slow the body. They didn't have antibiotics that, although welcome in emergencies, are often over-prescribed and upset the balance of flora in the intestine. There were no couch potatoes in pre-historic times, as the constant search for food required much walking, digging, and chasing. Stress was running away from a saber-toothed tiger, not divorce, bills, car pools, or a failing stock-market portfolio. And there was never enough food for our great grandparents to stuff themselves so that they could avoid feeling "stressed out." Nor would they have ignored the urge to defecate because they didn't like to use public bathrooms.

I'm not suggesting that we toss the niceties of life in the new millennium. However, I do believe that we must learn how to work, eat, drink, and act *with* our bodies rather than *despite* our bodies' design. We must work with our gut's beautiful design to achieve and maintain optimum health. Our guts are calling to us to listen to its message.

Throughout this book I have offered you valuable research and personal experience to assist you and your gut in a gut healing process. We all need support in making changes. In order to be successful in making new choices to befriend your gut, I encourage you to find a health practitioner, health coach, and/or body-mind therapist to support you as you take the journey to your gut's wisdom.

Remember: *You* have the power of choosing what foods, thoughts, and attitudes enter your gut and brain(s). Give yourself the gift of gut befriending choices. Your gut will thank you for it.

> Wisdom Blessings,
> Alyce M. Sorokie

The real voyage of discovery consists not in seeking new landscapes but in having new eyes.

> —Marcel Proust

∎ ∎ ∎ ∎ ∎ ∎ ∎ ∎ ∎

P.S. Well, I hope you've gotten to know me better and appreciate me as your friend and guide. We have a long, continuous journey ahead of us. For every step—big and small—that we take, I will be grateful. Be diligent and keep listening. Hopefully, I won't have to shout back at you too often. If you haven't noticed, I prefer to whisper.

> —Your Gut

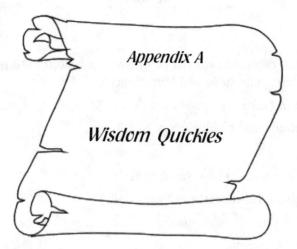

Appendix A

Wisdom Quickies

Abdominal Cramping/Spasms
▶ Warmth on belly.
▶ Belly breathe.
▶ Magnesium (500 mg).
▶ Belly massage.

Bad Breath
▶ Chlorophyll in water.
▶ Digestive enzyme.
▶ Colonic or enema.

Belching After Meals
▶ Enzyme with HCl with meals.

Constipation
▶ Belly breathe.
▶ Vitamin C (up to 5,000 mg).
▶ Fiber; drink morning and evening with extra water.
▶ Warmth on belly.
▶ Cascara sagrada or CKLS.
▶ Massage your belly.
▶ Digestive enzyme with meals.
▶ Colonic or enema.

Diarrhea

▸ Activated charcoal caps (three or four each hour until it subsides; remember: your stool will leave black).

▸ Bentonite (take recommended dosage).

▸ Acidophilus and bifidus every two hours.

Gas/Bloat

▸ Activated charcoal caps (as directed).

▸ Acidophilus/Bifidus (three times daily).

▸ Digestive enzyme with meals.

▸ Colonic or enema.

▸ Warmth on belly.

▸ Belly breathing.

▸ Stay off sugar.

Headache

▸ Warmth on belly.

▸ Belly breathe.

▸ Willowprin (natural aspirin).

▸ Omit possible trigger foods (food sensitivities, sugar, and caffeine).

▸ Colonic or enema (if headaches are a daily occurrence, check out leaky gut and constipation; headaches may be due to toxins in the system).

▸ Chamomile, peppermint, skullcap herb teas for tension headaches.

▸ Get a massage and relax.

Heartburn

▸ Immediately drink a full glass of water.

▸ Aloe vera juice.

▸ Liquid chlorophyll in water.

▸ Digestive enzymes with each meal.

Hemorrhoid Relief

▸ Bentonite or witch hazel (use a cotton ball to apply on hemorrhoids).

Irritable Bowel Syndrome

▶ Warmth on belly.

▶ Acidophilus and bifidus.

▶ Enteric-coated peppermint capsule (one to two caps, 20 minutes before meals).

▶ Belly breathe.

▶ Colonic or enema.

Just Stressed

▶ Belly breathe.

▶ Warmth on belly.

▶ Massage.

▶ Omit sugar, alcohol, and caffeine.

▶ Vitamin, mineral with extra Bs.

▶ Exercise.

Nausea

▶ Belly breathe.

▶ Ginger tea or capsules.

▶ Peppermint tea.

▶ Warmth on belly.

▶ Colonic or enema.

▶ Bentonite in water (three glasses, as directed).

▶ Multivitamin with vitamin B.

▶ Avoid sugar and carbohydrates.

PMS (crampy, bloated, irritated)

▶ Warmth on belly.

▶ Gentle stretches (yoga).

▶ Vitamin Bs.

▶ Primrose (200 mg for 10 days prior to menstrual flow).

▶ Keep bowels moving.

▶ Chamomile or peppermint tea.

▶ Stay off sugar, caffeine, and alcohol.

Skin Breakout

▶ Sauna.

▶ Apply bentonite to dry them up.

▶ Increase water.

▶ Acidophilus and bifidus daily.

▶ Cut out sugar and fried foods.

▶ Clear your bowels (colonic or enema).

Sugar Cravings

▶ Eat six small meals with protein (egg, tofu, chicken, fish, and nuts).

▶ Substitute fruit or dried fruit.

▶ Exercise.

▶ Get some "sweet" hugs.

▶ Colonic or enema.

Ulcer

▶ Aloe vera juice cools the pain.

▶ Belly breathe.

▶ Slippery elm tea.

▶ Relax.

Vegetable Deficiency

▶ Alfalfa tablets (six to eight tablets daily).

▶ Multivitamin and mineral tablet.

▶ Fresh vegetable juice.

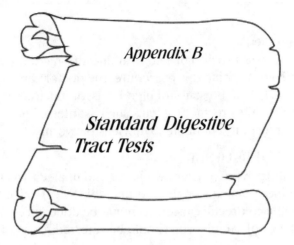

Appendix B

Standard Digestive Tract Tests

There are several digestive tract tests that can be used to detect and diagnose common gastrointestinal ailments. Discuss with your doctor the pros and cons of each test.

Barium Sulfate Test

Barium sulfate is used so that a technician can take X-ray studies of the digestive tract. Because barium is opaque to X-rays, your doctor can detect blockages, lesions, and other problems.

For an upper GI series, the patient swallows a barium "meal." The barium is then used to study the esophagus, stomach, and duodenum/small intestine.

For a lower GI series, a barium enema is given to the patient. This is to detect the presence of cancer or polyps in the colon.

Most doctors recommend the colonoscopy over a barium X-ray. Just a note about barium: It can dry out in the colon and become as hard as concrete so bowel movements may be harder to get back to normal. Colonics have served many in this case.

Endoscopy

A flexible, fiber-optic tube is introduced into the mouth and threaded through the esophagus, stomach, and the small bowel so that the doctor can make notes of lesions, blockages, inflammation, and other problems. He or she can also observe the liver and pancreatic duct systems and search for problems there.

Rectal Examinations

A doctor uses a proctoscope to examine the rectum (the lower five inches of the colon). Using this procedure, the doctor can inspect the mucous membrane for the presence of blood, pus, or mucus. The proctoscope can also identify other rectal problems such as internal hemorrhoids or a thread worm infection (commonly known as pinworms).

Fecal Occult Blood Test (FOBT)

Taken in the privacy of your own home and mailed to a lab for testing, this test examines a smear sample of your stool (feces) for hidden blood—a sign of possible colorectal cancer. It should be done once a year. If blood is found in the stool sample, you should be referred for a colonoscopy.

Sigmoidoscopy

A sigmoidoscopy is a brief, 10-minute procedure in which a sigmoidoscope, a hollow lighted tube, is inserted into the rectum. This allows the physician to examine the entire rectum and the lower portion of the large bowel.

A sigmoidoscopy is not a painful procedure. It can be performed in a doctor's office without anesthesia. However, the procedure may be slightly uncomfortable and embarrassing. (I recommended you try and overcome your embarrassment!)

It is best to have a cleansing enema an hour or two before the procedure. Otherwise, the physician will administer an enema about 15 minutes before the procedure. (Some doctors prefer that an enema not be used, as the liquid residue may obscure proper vision.)

After the sigmoidoscope is lubricated, it is gently inserted into the rectum. The doctor then introduces air via a bellows into the rectum so it is fully expanded for examination. Using the scope, the physician will be able to detect inflammation or tumor growth. He or she will also be able to take a biopsy of and subsequently remove polyps using an electrical current. The procedure takes about 10 minutes.

Colonoscopy

The colonoscope is a narrow, flexible, fiber-optic scope that is introduced into the rectum. Unlike a sigmoidoscope, a colonoscope enables your physician to examine the *entire* colon and the end of the small bowel. But like the sigmoidoscope, the colonoscope can also take biopsies and remove polyps or tumors.

A day or two before your colonoscopy, a bowel-cleansing medication may be prescribed. On the day of the colonoscopy, you may also receive an enema so that the doctor can better see the walls of the colon.

A colonoscopy may be performed in a doctor's office or in a hospital operating room. An hour before the colonoscopy, you'll get an intramuscular injection to make you feel relaxed and slightly sleepy. A small camera is attached to the colonoscope, and the doctor, as well as you, can view your large intestine. The colonoscope is then gently inserted into the rectum and threaded up through the bowel. This procedure is a little more extensive than the sigmoidoscopy.

A colonoscopy is considered much more thorough than a sigmoidoscopy. Katie Couric states, "Having a sigmoidoscopy is like only having one breast mammogramed." Check with your doctor and your "gut" and, based on your history, decide what would be the most advantageous.

Comprehensive Digestive Stool Analysis (CDSA)

CDSA is a valuable test, especially if you've tried everything and experimented with all the Gut Wisdom physical and emotional healing suggestions and your gut is still voicing its opinion (loudly!). CDSA gives you and your health practitioner valuable insight into what the heck is going on in your gut. It will give you information on bacterial imbalances and digestive functioning. The test is completed in the privacy of your own home.

The CDSA:

▷ Determines what possible harmful, disease-producing organisms are inhabiting your gut.

▷ Measures meats, vegetable fibers, and carbohydrates for digestibility.

▷ Checks fats for absorption.

▷ Measures stomach acid along with enzyme and bile levels (important for digestive and eliminative health).

▷ Reveals the level of friendly and unfriendly bacteria and the amount of yeast (candida), as well as any parasites that may be inhabiting your gut.

▷ Measures the predisposition for colon cancer.

▷ Most importantly, offers recommendations on how to correct imbalances.

CDSAs are recommended if you suffer from any of the following:

▹ Chronic indigestion.

▹ Chronic diarrhea or chronic, poorly formed stools.

▹ Colitis.

▹ Chronic constipation.

▹ Irritable bowel syndrome.

▹ Ulcers.

▹ Undigested food in stool.

▹ A suspicion of candida or parasites.

▹ Bloating.

▹ Skin problems (acne, psoriasis, eczema).

▹ Chronic fatigue.

▹ Chronic allergies or chronic sinus infections.

A CDSA is also recommended if you've been on Prednisone or any steroids for an extended period of time.

The CDSA helps you and your health practitioner with a comprehensive road map to your condition and what steps to take. (See Appendix C for phone numbers, or ask your health practitioner.)

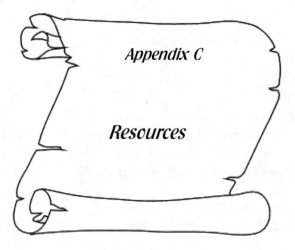

Appendix C

Resources

Gut Wisdom Cleanse Products

To order Gut Wisdom Cleanse products and all supplements mentioned in this book:

888–664–4732

www.gutwisdom.com

Belly Buddy

888–664–4732

www.gutwisdom.com

Anti-Parasite Products

Awareness Corporation

Orders: 800–69–AWARE

Sponsor #2446301

Discounts available for distributors

STOCK #

1132	Clear™ Parasite Cleanse (30 caps)	$27.95
1352	Clear™ Parasite Cleanse (90 caps)	$69.95
1122	Experience™	$39.95

Laboratories for Detoxification Testing and Assessment

Comprehensive Digestive Stool Analysis (CDSA) and Parasite Testing

Contact:

Great Smokies Diagnostic Laboratory

63 Zillicoa St.

Asheville, NC 28801

800–522–4762

Meridian Valley Clinical Laboratory
24030 132nd Ave. S.E.
Kent, WA 98042
800–234–6825

Holistic Health Organizations

Contact these organizations for practitioners in your area to help assist you with gut healing and befriending journey.

I-ACT (International Association of Colon Therapists)
PO Box 461285
San Antonio, TX 78245-1285
210–366–2888
i-act.org

Partners in Wellness
1967 N. Dayton
Chicago, IL 60614
773–868–4062
www.gutwisdom.com

American Holistic Medical Association
6728 Old McLean Village Dr.
McLean, VA 22101
703–556–9728

American Association of Naturopathic Physicians
601 Valley St., #105
Seattle, WA 98109
202–298–0125

American Association of Acupuncture and Oriental Medicine
433 Front St.
Catasauqua, PA 18032
610–433–2448

American Massage Therapy Association
820 Davis St., #100
Evanston, IL 60201-4444
847–864–0123

The American Metabolic Institute
180 Otay Lakes Rd., #107
Bonita, CA 91902
William R. Fry, Director
800–388–1083
ami-health.com
E-mail: ami@beat-cancer.com

Alternative Cancer Therapies
The Cancer Control Society
2043 N. Berendo St.
Los Angeles, CA 91902
323–663–7801

American Natural Hygiene Society
PO Box 30630
Tampa, FL 33630
anhs.org

Books on diet and nutrition. Call for health magazine and subscription (alternative healing).

A.R.E. (Association for Research and Enlightenment)
67th St. & Atlantic Ave.
Virginia Beach, VA 23451
804–428–3588

Cookbooks With Gut-Friendly Recipes

Gluten Free Kitchen by Robin Ryberg

Gluten Free Gourmet Cooks Fast and Healthy by Bette Hagman

Cleanse Cookbook by Christine Dreher

Vegetarian Cooking for Those with Allergies by Raphael Rettner, D.C.

Magazines

Living Without
www.livingwithout.com
847–480–8810

An informative magazine that offers inspiring stories and recipes on wheat-free and gluten-free living.

Recommended Reading Material

The Second Brain by Michael Gershon, M.D. (Perennial, 2000).

Molecules of Emotion by Candace Pert, Ph.D. (Scribner, 1997).

The Complete Book of Chinese Health and Healing by Daniel Reid (Shambala, 1995).

The Power of the Mind to Heal by Joan Borysenko, Ph.D. (HayHouse, Inc., 1994).

Back to Eden by Jethro Kloss (Lotus Press, 1999).

Your Body Believes Every Word You Say by Barbara Hoberman Levine (Aslan Publishing, 1991).

Want to Go Away to Cleanse and Get Your Gut on Track?

Optimum Health Institute of San Diego
6970 Central Ave.
Lemon Grove, CA 91945
616–464–3346

Offers healthy programs focusing body-mind detoxification that include wheat grass juice, raw foods, colon therapy, enemas, and massage.

Optimum Health Institute of Texas
265 Cedar Lane
Cedar Creek, TX 78612
512–303–4817

Offers healthy programs focusing body-mind detoxification that include raw wheat grass juice, foods, colon therapy, enemas, massage.

We Care Health Retreat
18000 Long Canyon Rd.
Desert Hot Springs, CA 92241
800–888–2523

Offers fasting programs with specific cleansing products, colon therapy, massage, yoga, and hot mineral baths.

Kripalu Center for Yoga and Health
Box 1793
Lenox, MA 1240
413–637–3280

Retreats, classes, and medical evaluations.

Gut Wisdom Speaking Engagements and Workshops

For updated information about Gut Wisdom Cleanses, classes, and workshops, please visit *www.gutwisdom.com.*

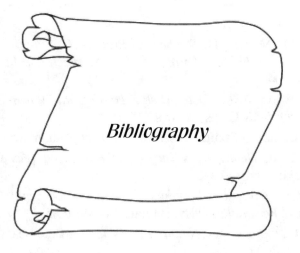

Bibliography

Andrews, Ted. *The Healer's Manual: A Beginner's Guide to Vibrational Therapies.* Llewellyn Publications, Revised Edition, 1988.

Balch, M.D., Jamie F. and Phyllis A. Balch, C.N.C. *Prescription for Nutritional Healing.* Avery Penguin Putnam, 1997.

Barry, Linda and Jan Fawcett. *Internal Cleansing: Rid Your Body of Toxins to Naturally and Effectively Fight Heart Disease, Chronic Pain, Fatigue, PMS, Menopause Symptoms and More.* Prima Publishing, 2nd Revised Edition, 2000.

Batmangheidj, M.D., F. *Your Body's Many Cries for Water.* Tagman Press, 1996.

Bland, Ph.D., Jeffery. *Digestive Enzymes.* McGraw Hill—NTC, 1983.

———. *Intestinal Toxicity and Inner Cleansing.* McGraw Hill/ Contemporary Books, 1989.

Colbin, Annmarie. *Food & Healing.* Ballantine Books (trade paper), Reissue Edition, 1996.

Condron, Daniel R. and David C. McKnight. *Permanent Healing.* SOM Pub & Production, 1993.

Cornell, Ph.D., Ann Weiser. *The Power of Focusing.* MJF Books, Reprint Edition, 1999.

Gates, Donna. *The Body Ecology Diet.* BED Publishers, 2002.

Genen, Ruth. *When Food is Love.* Plane, a Division of the Perguen Group, 1991.

Gershon, M.D., Michael D. *The Second Brain: A Groundbreaking New Understanding of Nervous Disorders of the Stomach and Intestine.* Perennial, 2000.

Hass, M.D., Elson M. *The Detox Diet: A How-To and When-To Guide to Cleansing the Body.* Celestial Arts, 1996.

——— and Cameron Stauth. *The False Fat Diet.* Ballantine Books, 2001.

Heinerman, John. *Heinerman's Encyclopedia of Juices, Teas & Tonics.* Prentice Hall Trade, 1996.

Hendricks, Guy. *Conscious Breathing: Breathwork for Health, Stress Release, and Personal Mastery.* Bantam Books, 1995.

Hobbs, L.A.C., Christopher. *Natural Liver Therapy.* Botanica, 2nd Edition, 2000.

Hoffman, M.D., Ronald. *Seven Weeks to a Settled Stomach.* Pocket Books, Reissue Edition, 1991.

Hunter, Beatrice Trum. *Gluten Intolerance.* McGraw-Hill/Contemporary Books, 1999.

Jaakkimainen, S. E. and J. Bombardier. *Risk for Seniors Gastrointestinal Complaints Related to Use of Nonsteroidal Anti-Inflammatory Drugs.* Annals of Internal Medicine, 1991.

Jensen, Ph.D., Bernard. *Patient Education Chart of the Bowel Reflex Points.* Bernard Jensen Research Institute, Copyright 1992.

———.*Tissue Cleansing Through Bowel Management.* Avery Penguin Putnam, 1981.

Keller, Jeanne. *Healing With Water: Special Applications and Uses of Water in Home Remedies for Everyday Ailments.* Prentice Hall, 1983.

Kellogg, M.D., John Harvey. *The Crippled Colon.* The Modern Medicine Publishing Co., 1931.

Lappe, Marc. *When Antibiotics Fail: Restoring the Ecology of the Body.* North Allontic Books, 1986.

Lipski, M.S., C.C.N., Elizabeth and Jeffery S. Bland. *Digestive Wellness.* McGraw-Hill/Contemporary Books, 2nd Edition, 1999.

Lowell, Jax Peters. *Against the Grain: The Slightly Eccentric Guide to Living Well Without Gluten or Wheat.* Henry Holt (paper), Reprint Edition, 1996.

Mindell, Earl. *Mindell's Vitamin Bible for the 21st Century.* Warner Books, Reissue Edition, 1999.

Murray, Michael and Joseph Pizzorno. *Encyclopedia of Natural Medicine*. Prima Publishing, 1991.

Myss, Caroline and C. Norman Shealy. *The Creation of Health: The Emotional, Psychological and Spiritual Responses That Promote Health and Healing*. Three Rivers Press, Reprint Edition, 1998.

Padus, Emrika. *Complete Guide to Your Emotions and Your Health: Hundreds of Proven Techniques to Harmonize Mind and Body for Happy, Healthy Living*. Rodale Press, Revised Edition, 1992.

Page, N.D., Ph.D. and Linda Rector. *Healthy Healing—A Guide to Self-Healing for Everyone*. Healthy Healing Publishers, 11th Edition, 2000.

Rosenthal, Sara M. *50 Ways to Prevent Colon Cancer*. McGraw-Hill/Contemporary Books.

Saltzman, Allen. *The Belly and Its Power*. Yoga Tools, 1987.

Scala, Dr., James. *Eating Right for a Bad Gut: The Complete Nutritional Guide to Ileitis, Colitis, Crohn's Disease and Inflammatory Bowel Disease*. Plume, Reprint Edition, 1992.

Shahani, K. M. and B. A. Friend. "Nutritional and Therapeutic Aspect of Lactobacelli". *Journal of Applied Nutrition*, 1973.

Shock, Lisa S. and Dr. Robert Erdmann. *Food Cravings*. Apple Pub Co., Ltd., 1999.

Teeguarden, Iona Marsaa. *The Joy of Felling, Bodymind Acupressure*. Japan Publications, 4th Printing, 1994.

Trenev, Natasha. *Probiotics: Nature's Internal Healers*. Avery Penguin Putnam, 1998.

Van Auken, John. *Edgar Cayce's Approach to Rejuvenation of the Body*. A.R.E. Press, 1997.

Wald, Ken Dycht. *Body-Mind*. Putman Bertey Group, Inc., 1997.

Walker, Dr. Norman W. *Colon Health Key to Vibrant Life*. Norwalk Press, 1979.

Webster, David. *Intestine Gardening*. Excerpts from the writings of Dr. James Eprisingham, D.Sc., Ph.D.

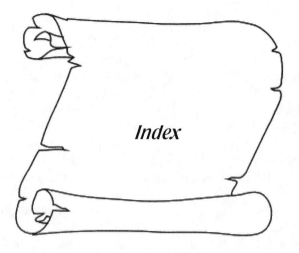

Index

A

acid and alkaline balance in body, 66
acidophilus, 92-95
  and gut cleansing, 159
alcohol, negative effects of, 86, 121
alkaline and acid balance in body, 66
allergies to food, 67
amino acids, 74, 78
amylase, 39
antacids, negative effects of,
  116-118
antibiotics, 113-114
  in eggs, 75
  and friendly bacteria, 113-114
  in meat products, 113
antioxidants, 70, 74
appendix, digestive process and,
  41-42
arachidonic acid, 76
autointoxication, 44, 52-54, 134
autonomic nervous system, 25-26

B

bacteria
  and antibodies in saliva, 36
  and gut cleansing, 152-154
  and lymphocytes, 40
  and maintaining a balance with
  fiber, 91
  festering in colon, 53
  killed off by antibiotics, 113
bacteria,
  unfriendly, 42-43, 50-51
  friendly, 42-43, 50, 92-95
  large intestine and, 42-43
  sugar and unfriendly, 84, 121
ballooning of colon, 56
belly breathing, 124
  and gut cleansing, 158
belly massage, 128-130
  and gut cleansing, 158
belly, *see gut.*
benzodiazepines, 18
bifido bacterium, *see bifidus.*
bifidobacteria, *see bifidus.*
bifidus, 50, 92-95
  and gut cleansing, 159
bile and the gall bladder, 46-47

bioflavonoids, 71
Bodymind, 118
bowel movements,
    functional, 57-58
        characteristis of, 58
    normal rhythm of, 116-117
    squatting and, 139
    tracking transit time of, 117-118
bowel problems and traveling,
    223-228
breathing, 124-126
    deep, 30, 32-33
brushing, dry skin, 130
    and gut cleansing, 157
Burkett, Dennis, 91

C

caffeine and gut health, 82-84
calcium, 76, 79
    depleted by coffee, 121
cancer,
    alcohol and, 86
    colon, 11-12, 19, 56, 216-217, 220
        explanation, causes, and
            treatment of, 216-223
    colorectal, 19, 216-217, 220
        statistics about, 19
    rectal, 19
    urethra, 12
cancer-fighting substances, 70
candida albanicans, *see candida*.
candida, 51-52, 73, 85-86, 93, 134
    explanation, causes, and
        treatment of, 178-184
    steroids and, 113
    antibiotics and, 113
carcinogens,
    binding with fiber, 91
    source of, 51-52
castor oil packs, 142-143
    and gut cleansing, 157

Cayce, Edgar, 142
central nervous system, 25-26
Cheskin, Lawrence, 97
Chi Nei Tsong, 119-120
Chia, Maneewan, 119-120
Chia, Mantak, 119-120
chlorophyll,
    benefits of, 73
    gut cleansing and, 160
cholesterol and eggs, 75
cholesterol, effects of fiber on, 91
chyme, 37-39, 41
Clayton Naturopathic College, 14
cleansing the gut, 151-169
colitis, 58, 68, 79
Colon Health, 41
colon
    and gut cleansing, 152-154
    and reflex points, 136
    cancer, 11-12, 19, 56, 216-217, 220
        explanation, causes, and
            treatment of, 216-223
        risk factors for, 51
    hydrotherapy, 133-138
    therapy, 13
        and detoxification, 135
        and gut cleansing, 157
colon,
    ballooning of, 56
    dysfunction of, 50, 54-57
    problems beginning in, 49-50
    spastic, 201
colonics, 132-138
colorectal cancer, 19, 216-217, 220
colostomies, 19
comfort foods and gut ailments, 62
constipation,
    explanation, causes, and
        treatment of, 172-178
    statistics about, 19
Crohn's disease, 68, 79

D

dairy products
  and digestive health, 78-79
  and lactase enzyme, 93
dairy products,
  combining with other foods,
  99-100
  friendly, 102
detox baths, 131-132
  and gut cleansing, 157
detoxification and colon therapy,
  135
diaphragm, digestion process and,
  47-48
diarrhea,
  explanation, causes, and
  treatment of, 184-188
  traveling and, 225
Diet, the Gut Wisdom, 108-110
digestive enzymes,
  produced in pancreas, 39
  using with meals, 95-98
digestive process, 35-48
  balance of, 48
  diaphragm and solar plexus and,
  47-48
  the mouth and, 36-37
  immune protectors and, 40
  secretory IgA [S(IgA)] and, 41
  the appendix and, 41-42
  the gall bladder and, 46-47
  the large intestine and, 42-43
  the liver and, 43-46
  the pancreas and, 39-40
  the small intestine and, 38-39
  the stomach and, 37-38
Digestive Wellness, 77
diverticuli, 53
diverticulitis, 188

diverticulosis, 55
  explanation, causes, and
  treatment of, 188-192
  statistics about, 19
dybosis, 50-52
Dychtwald, Ken, 118

E

Eat Right or Die Young, 28
E-coli, 94
emotions
  and irritable bowel syndrome, 32
  and physical responses, 27-28
endorphins, 29
enemas, 132-134, 138-139
energy system, 25, 29-30
enteric nervous system, 17-18, 25-27
enzymes
  in foods, 97
  in saliva, 36
  needed for digestion, 95-98
essential fatty acids, 81-82
exercise, 140-142

F

fat,
  friendly (natural), 81
  hydrogenated, 80
  products low in, 81
  saturated, 80-81
fiber, 71-72
  and beans, 78
fiber, health functions of, 91-92
fight or flight response, 26
food and gut-befriending gestures,
  69-100
  alcohol, 86-87
  beans and fiber, 78
  being selective about fish, 77-78
  caffeine, 82-84
  digestive enzyme, 95-98

eggs, 75-76
fats, hydrogenated and saturated, 80-82
fiber, 91-92
exploring grains, 69-70
friendly bacteria, 92-95
fruit servings, 71-72
juices, 72-74
nuts and seeds, 74-75
processed foods, 88
red meat vs. poultry, fish, and soy, 76-77
soft drinks, 87-88
soy, rice, and cultured products vs. dairy, 78-79
sugar, 84-86
veggie servings, 70-71
water intake, 89-90
wisdom food combining, 98-100
food
   allergies and sensitivities, 67-69
      detecting, 69
   overindulgence, 121
food,
   effects of unfriendly, 66
   friendly and foe, 65-69
   proper combination of, 98-100
      chart of, 100
      diet including, 108-110
Freedom from Stress, 125
fruit juices, 72-74
fruits,
   combining with other foods, 99-100
   friendly, 101
   gut-friendly, 71-72
fungus in gut, 51-52

G

gall bladder, digestion process and, 46-47
gall stones,
   treating, 73
   preventing, 74
gas, bloating, and belching, 197
gastric reflux, 196
gastrointestinal problems in United States, 19
Gershon, Michael, 25, 116
Getting Well Again, 63
gluten, 69-70
grains, friendly, 101
Guide to Colon Health, 96
gut ailments,
   how we create, 30-31
   comfort foods and, 62
gut and
   candida, 178-184
   castor oil packs, 142-143
   colon cancer, 216-223
   connection with cerebral brain, 25, 128
   constipation, 172-178
   desire for awareness, 60-62
   diarrhea, 184-188, 225
   diverticulosis, 188-192
   hemorrhoids, 193-195
   indigestion, 195-201
   irritable bowel syndrome, 201-205
   lactose intolerance, 205-207
   movement and exercise, 140-142
   parasites, 207-211
   traveling, 223-228
   ulcers, 211-216
   warmth, 126-127
Gut Associated Lymph Tissues (GALT), 40

gut befrienders, creating a functional relationship with, 123-149
gut health
  and forgiveness, 144-145
  and journaling, 143
  and toxic thoughts and feelings, 118-119
Gut Wisdom Cleanse, 151-169
gut
  exploration exercises, 30
  massage, 30
gut,
  bacteria in, 50
  building relationship with, 31-33
  embracing discomfort and conversations with, 146-149
  immune cells in, 28
  listening to your, 23-24
  messages from, 15-16, 62
  organisms that affect health of, 51-52
  parasites in, 52
  psychological stress and, 17
  recognizing importance of, 16-17
  results of emotional disturbances on, 29
  symptoms of, 20
  things that affect health of, 14
  undigested emotions in, 119-120
gut-befriending food gestures, 69-100
gut-brain, 17-18, 25

H

Hay, Louise, 212
heartburn, 195-196
hemorrhoids, explanation, causes, and treatment of, 193-195
Hendricks Body/Mind Centering Process, 14

hernia, hiatal, 196-197
Houston, Jean, 30
H-pylori, 94
hydrochloric acid in stomach, 96-97
hydrotherapy, 131-132
  colon, 133

I

IBS, *see irritable bowel syndrome.*
immune
  cells in gut, 28
  protectors in digestive tract, 40
indigestion, explanation, causes, and treatment of, 195-201
  gas, bloating, and belching, 197
  gastric reflux, 196
  heartburn, 195-196
  hiatal hernia, 196-197
Ingram, Cass, 28
insulin and the pancreas, 39
intestine,
  large, digestive process and, 42-43
  small, digestive process and, 38-39
irritable bowel syndrome (IBS), explanation, causes, and treatment of, 201-205
irritable bowel syndrome, 56
  and dairy, 79
  and emotion, 32
  statistics, 19

J

Jensen, Bernard, 54, 95
journaling
  and gut cleansing, 158
  and gut health, 143

K

Kellogg, J.H., 133

L

lactase, 93
lactobacillus acidophilus, *see*
  acidophilus.
lactose intolerance, explanation,
  causes, and treatment of,
  205-207
large intestine, digestive process
  and, 42-43
laxatives,
  getting off of, 225-226
  negative effects of, 114-115
lipase, 39
Lipski, Elizabeth, 77
liver,
  cleansing, 73
  digestion process and, 43-46
Love, Medicine and Miracles, 144
lymphocytes, 40

M

magnesium, 76
massage, belly, 128-130
  and gut cleansing, 158
Mind Body Connection, The, 48
Molecules of Emotion, 27-28, 60, 128
moods and eating, 121-122
MSG, 88

N

neurogastroenterology, 17-18
neuropeptides, 18, 25, 27-28
nonsteroidal anti-inflammatory
  drugs (NSAIDs), 112
Norenberger, Phil, 125
Northrup, Christiane, 36
NSAIDs, *see nonsteroidal anti-*
  inflammatory drugs

O

omega-3, 77, 81-82
omega-6, 81-82
organs, role of internal, 36
osteoporosis, 76

P

pancreas, digestive process and,
  39-40
parasites, 52
  explanation, causes, and
  treatment of, 207-211
parasympathetic nervous system, 26
Partners in Wellness, 16
Percival, Mark, 48
Pert, Candace, 27-28, 60, 128
pinworm, 208
prolapsus, 55
prostaglandin, 37, 81-82, 112-113
protease, 39
proteins, combining with other
  foods, 99-100
ptyalin, 36
putrefaction, 52
  and inhibited enzyme production,
  96-97
  and red meat, 76
  and soda, 88
  and sugar, 84, 121

R

reflex points and colon, 136
roundworm, 208

S

S(IgA), *see secretory IgA*.
saliva,
  antibodies in, 36
  enzymes in, 36
secretory IgA [S(IgA)], 41, 119-120
Siegal, Bernie, 144

Simonton, Carl, 63
Simonton, Stephanie, 63
skin brushing, dry, 130
    and gut cleansing, 157
small intestine, digestive process
    and, 38-39
solar plexus, digestion process and,
    47-48
squat, wisdom, 139
starches, combining with other
    foods, 99-100
steroids, 112-113
stomach, digestive process and,
    37-38
sugars, negative effects of excess,
    84-85
sympathetic nervous system, 26

T
Tenney, Louise, 96
The Second Brain, 25, 116
*Tissue Cleansing Through Bowel
    Management*, 18, 54
toxic thoughts and feelings, 118-119
toxins
    and antibodies in saliva, 36
    and gut cleansing, 152-154
    and parasites, 208
    and the liver, 44-45
    from colon, 53
    releasing through skin, 130
toxins,
    neutralizing, 73
    symptoms caused by, 57
trauma and effect on gut, 31
traveling and your bowels, 223-228

U
U.S. Department of Health and
    Human Services, 19
ulcer,
    explanation, causes, and
    treatment of, 211-216
    healing, 73
    increased risk of, 112

V
Valium, 18
vegetable juices, 72-73
    and gut cleansing, 160
vegetables,
    combining with other foods,
    99-100
        friendly, 101
        gut-friendly, 70-71
vitamin C, healing properties of, 71

W
Walker, Morton, 133
Walker, Norman, 41, 49
warmth and gut cleansing, 158
water,
    healing with, 131-132
    health functions of, 89-90
wheat grass, 73
    and gut cleansing, 160
wisdom-cises, 140-142
Women's Bodies, Women's Wisdom,
    36

X
Xanax, 18

Y
You Can Heal Your Life, 212

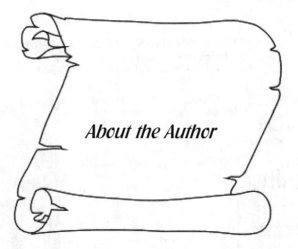

About the Author

ALYCE M. SOROKIE has been marinating in alternative health ever since she can remember. Raised in the 1950s by parents who were pioneers in the holistic field in Chicago, Alyce continues to study and integrate alternative healing modalities. She resides in Chicago. She is the founder of Partners in Wellness, a holistic clinic specializing in colon therapy in Chicago's infamous Lincoln Park area. Alyce has been a digestive consultant and C.T. for 18 years. As one of the area's foremost authorities on topics of gut digestion and the relationship of stress-to-gut health, she is the facilitator of Gut Wisdom workshops, classes, and cleanses. She is also the creator of the Belly Buddy, an aromatic, heatable pillow sold nationally. Featured in the *Chicago Tribune* and the *New York Times,* she is passionate about teaching people how to learn to listen to the gut's "voice" and empowering them to make choices that are more health-minded.

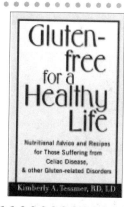
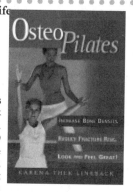
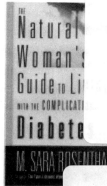
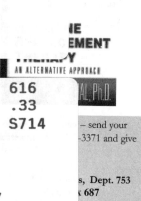